Without Utterance:
Tales from the Other Side of Language

Without Utterance:

Tales from the Other Side of Language

Copyright © Ruth Codier Resch

Parts of this memoir have been previously published in *Topics in Stroke Rehabilitation*, "The Lost Adulthood" and in www.persimmontree.org "Through the Eyes...."

Cover and Interior art by Ruth Codier Resch

ISBN-13: 978-0-9837422-7-2

Resch, Ruth Codier
Without Utterance: Tales from the Other Side of Language/
Ruth Codier Resch

Library of Congress Control Number: 2012945637

First Edition: September 2012

Printed in the United States of America,
the United Kingdom and Australia

0 9 8 7 6 5 4 3 2 1

Starseed Publications,
2204 E Grand Ave.
Everett, WA 98201

Without Utterance:
Tales from the Other Side of Language

Ruth Codier Resch

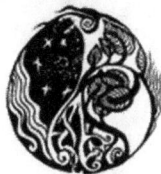

Starseed Publications,
2204 E Grand Ave.
Everett, WA 98201

For:

Rachael

Richard

Martha

We must be willing to give up the life
we've planned, in order to have the life
that is waiting for us.

Joseph Campbell

...to be human
is to become visible
while carrying
what is hidden
as a gift to others...

David Whyte

TABLE OF CONTENTS

LIST OF ILLUSTRATIONS

Foreword
Paradigm Shift

Martha Taylor Sarno, M.A., M.D. honoris causa
Research Professor, Department of Rehabilitation Medicine
NYU School of Medicine, New York City, September 2012

Until quite recently, little thought has been given to the subjective experience of living with aphasia. Yet, from the perspective of the person with aphasia its emergence is not just an acute, traumatic event but is felt in all of life's dimensions in unique and unpredictable ways rather than in a sequence of stages. Living with aphasia is a process of transition and transformation. Aphasia not only disconnects the person from the community but invariably alters the person's identity and sense of self. Living effectively with aphasia requires an evolving 'self'' and a transition from one 'self' to another as the self is reconstructed.

Many of the issues faced by those who manage the rehabilitation of persons with aphasia stem from its dependence on a medical model which predictably focuses on pathology. This model has abandoned long-term quality of life issues and served to further "medicalize" the management of persons with aphasia beyond the acute stage. The long term consequences of aphasia cannot be solved in today's medical environment.

Ruth Resch's rich description of her life with aphasia over three decades is a testament to the necessity of our understanding the 'insider' perspective. Her earlier career as a psychoanalyst and researcher of babies and mothers endowed her with a deep understanding of the development of the inner self and the capacity of the sensory systems to bring balance and fulfillment across the life span. After suffering a stroke and the onset of aphasia she engaged successfully in the difficult process of separating the 'verbal mind' from the visual mind, thereby providing a platform for arousing previously enjoyed pleasures in painting, drawing, and music.

These evolved as places of rest and avenues of healing fulfillment. As a person with aphasia she found no comparable equivalent in the world of words.

Her expression through art translated into a feeling of balance, an adaptation through the creation of pleasure, which she views as central to the life of recovery.

Dr. Resch describes her quest for meaningfulness in all aspects of daily life and how she has learned to use the environment as a source of fulfillment and well being. Her ability to connect with the ever-changing natural environment has provided easy access to a stimulating non-verbal world.

Readers at all levels, patients, students, and clinicians, will gain a deeper understanding of the inner life of someone with aphasia. We are grateful to Dr. Resch for sharing her innermost feelings in describing her long journey in the quest for a new life. Her courage, integrity, and passion for the human spirit are an inspiration to us all.

Art as Brain Recovery

Andrea Gellin Shindler
Founder Executive Director, Foundation for Human Potential,
Chicago, IL.

Having learned of Ruth Resch's extraordinary story and work from Dr. Martha Taylor Sarno, I was immediately taken by her remarkable artwork, in the face of stroke-related, brain damage.

Ruth Resch was and is a fighter, determined to communicate in the best way possible, showing that artistic expression is her mode.

Having had experience with a young female patient, years ago, who had had a similar experience, I developed the Foundation for Human Potential to share the influence of alternative means of communication, in so doing, advocating strongly for the arts/artistic expression — a most positive channel for rehabilitation.

Books from prominent authors which have developed to support the notion that positive rehabilitation is an ongoing process, include: Begley, S. Train Your Brain, Change Your Mind; Schwartz, M., Begley, S. The Mind and the Brain: Neuroplasticity and the Power of Mental Force; Doidge, N. The Brain the Changes Itself; LeDoux, J. The Emotional Brain; Caplan, L. Striking Back at Stroke.

Bravo to Ruth Resch for teaching the world that rehabilitation can be an idiosyncratic development, to which close attention must be paid. Positive options for rehabilitation will, thereby, ensue for the betterment of rehabilitation for all individuals.

www.fhponline.org

Perspectives on Identity and Self

Howard B. Levine, M.D.
Psychoanalyst and Faculty of the Psychoanalytic Institute of
New England East

Uttering a word is like striking a note on the keyboard of the imagination,"' Ludwig Wittgenstein once wrote . Infants come into the world ready and equipped for language. And words, those essential elements that help make up a language, become markers and the building blocks of who we are... to ourselves, to others.

There is something about language, our capacity for words, which forms and reflects the in-born, in-built grammar of our being, the scaffolding of our self. Language emerges naturally from our earliest and most cherished relationships - what will become and we will call our mother tongue. It orders our universe and constructs our very selves and our places within that universe.

In the privacy of our own minds, regardless of how much schooling we may have, we are, each of us, spinners of narrative, weavers of words, bards of our own existence. We are creating, each in our own personal and particular way, our sense of self and our world, and then created in the minds of others. The binding power of words are the notes arising from the keyboard of our imagination.

But what if that instrument is damaged -- keys missing, hollow, or ringing false? Worse yet, what if strings are torn, frame shattered, the very scaffolding gone wrong, gone very wrong? Aphasia! Absence of language. What if the vital link is sundered between inside and outside, sensation and meaning, emotion and intellect, self and other? The loss of self, of competence of community, the sense of shame and isolation, may be unbearable.

William James had it that the world was a 'blooming, buzzing confusion' ordered and made tolerable by filtering through our senses. Freud and later Wilfred Bion, the English psychoanalyst, believed that it was through the agency and action of language, words, that this filtration process occurred.

For Freud, the memory trace of the sensuous sound of the word, tied to the emotional quality of the relationship with the earliest caregivers, made the otherwise unbearable frustration of absence tolerable. This bond was the origin of the development of the psyche, a beginning sense of self and meaning. If raw sensory experience is in its self too much to bear, words and language were the keys to containing its onslaught and making it bearable.

For Bion, it is language as narrative and its relation to pictorial representation, the capacity to dream even when awake, that helps detoxify the otherwise assaultive, even traumatic, sensory experience of being in the world. Words, said and heard, in their structuring role in the human psyche turns the onslaught into something we can come to know, to tolerate, to reflect upon. They ultimately come to make us feel what we believe ourselves to be.

Without Utterance is an astonishing story of human courage, resilience and discovery. I first met Ruth Resch prior to her stroke when she was a young and vibrant professional woman, gifted as a teacher, writer and therapist, a psychologist entering the fullness of her creativity. We were colleagues and became good friends. Life's circumstances intervened, we saw each other only occasionally and then one day I received a phone call telling me that she had had a stroke. A dissecting aneurysm of the artery that supplied the speech area of her brain had suddenly torn her away from words, language and all meaning that they might convey. Without words, without language, the very essence of her being was altered. She not only lost the ability to express her thoughts and meanings – she suffered "expressive aphasia," while thankfully her capacity to understand remained intact - but she discovered that the very grid with which we unthinkingly order the world was changed, even shattered. As Ruth has put it, "The continuous arc of personal narrative and the continual construction of a sense of self, …. The essence of my very being is altered" (p. 12).

The human cortex is organized in two separate hemispheres linked together and integrated by an extensive network of connections. The left side of the brain, where speech is located, serves intellect, logic and rationality. The right organizes passion, emotion and aesthetic pursuits. Ordinarily, we take the coupling of the two sides of the brain for granted. Intellect and emotion; speech and aesthetic form; language and art. The integration and stratification of these disparate modes of sensation, experience and being is the stuff of ordinary infant development.

Ironically, Ruth Resch's career was centered on the study and treatment of the pre-verbal infant. The child before language and the difficulties in forming attachments and relationships that are associated with autism and other forms of pervasive developmental disorders.

 Now, all bets were off. "When I lost so much of my expressive verbal mind, I lost part of the subtle behavioral syntax attached to it." (p. 58). Even more, as she later wrote to me: "Loss of language at best eclipses the self. At worst it makes for invisibility and isolation in the social sphere, annihilation.... If you don't speak, you are not there."

If she was to recover, Ruth's very world and knowing how to be in it had to be re-ordered. It was all ground that once easily won in childhood, had now to be painfully re-conquered. "In losing language, I also lost how language connects me to intention and planning in my life, unhinging ordinary parts of my daily life." (p. 58). "It used to be so simple to make words and have feelings at the same time. My halting words now are too gossamer to shelter the mass of sensation and emotion underneath the enduring calamities of my day." (p. 27).

And yet, to her surprise and even delight, she discovered that there were unexpected opportunities in this chaos. It is a truism that all knowledge is a two-edged sword. The known and the expected are powerful organizers and filters of experience. We are so deeply embedded in our pre-conceptions and language dependent ways of organizing the world and our experience of it that we have great difficulty in letting anything evolve in a truly novel and unexpected context. Order tends to create expectation and shape observation, almost pre-selecting what may come to be seen. Bion once said that in order to discover something truly novel, we may have to view it in 'a beam of intense darkness' so that we are not blinded by the light of what we already know and believe to be so.

Chaos, as disturbing as it can be, can also breed opportunity. Freed from words and language, forced to rebuild the world within a new balance of sensory modalities, new shapes may form and relationships may be seen that were hidden before by the known and the expected. New ways of ordering things, new relationships between otherwise familiar elements may emerge.

As words slowly began to return, finding herself easily exhausted by left brain activity – reading, writing, talking to patients – Ruth discovered that her stamina for art and music increased. A new world opened up to her; not just as she began to study art, but as she discovered the freedom that comes from a change in the balance of how she existed in and experienced the world around her. "I begin to see and feel more and more the life force around me, more perceptive to the sentience I have never before seen and to the sensory languages I've never heard." (p. 73).

Even more powerfully, she discovered that "I am moving further and further in the direction of living in sensory and non-verbal worlds. The wealth of sensation, reception, and communication in the unconscious meets the conscious brain's aptitudes to walk in other worlds, to know altered states of mind, and to be in service in different ways, without so many words." (p. 59, italics added).

So began a journey, not only of recovery, but deep spiritual discovery in ways that were unexpected, deeply personal and powerfully transformative. A journey towards new ways of being; being in the world, experiencing that world, experiencing one's self in the world, "experiencing new languages not given by words or sometimes even by communicative sounds. These non-verbal languages are sensory syntax, sensory language, felt though my body." (p. 88).

Beyond the personal courage and heroism, beyond the testament to life force and human resilience, this is a story of deep spiritual meaning and metaphysical import: of seeing and being; of encounter and discovery. And it is an attempt to give hope and voice to the many who remain speechless.

In asking me to write this Foreword, Ruth said, "Making the book a reality now, crosses a huge boundary for me-- stepping into public articulate visibility. Visibility for myself, but as much for the hundreds of thousands of people with aphasia who cannot tell their story. Speaking is a gift, a complex, mind/body gorgeous miracle. We should be speaking carefully and be on our knees in gratitude."

Indeed, as we are grateful to Ruth for this book. As she has written: "Without the landscape of utterance, I've unearthed treasures, wreathed and adorned myself with an extravagance of sensory languages. Dressed in them, I've gone to the heart of what is ... and pressed toward the edges of what can be. I've moved in spaces where mystery collides with mind and melts into vision." (p. 140).

The Mystical Life

David Spangler
Author, Mystic and Spiritual Teacher

It's not easy to define the life of a mystic. Mystics come in so many different flavors and expressions, living a wide variety of lifestyles and following diverse spiritual paths or even at times no overt spiritual path at all. The popular image is that of someone divorced from the concerns and tribulations of the world, spending his or her time in deep communion with the Sacred, and floating about on clouds of otherworldly bliss. Even a cursory study of the lives of many famous mystics shows how unrepresentative and even ludicrous such an image is. Yes, these individuals did experience a deep union of soul and sacred, but most of them were hardly otherworldly. They were involved with the people and events around them, and many of them were deeply engaged in social movements seeking justice for the dispossessed of their time in history. They were moved by a deep conviction of compassion.

It is true that most of the mystics of whom we are most aware lived and worked within a religious context, so it's not surprising that we think of mysticism as a profession for spiritual people, people who have felt a calling to a religious life. But anyone can be a mystic, for at the heart of the mystical life is a simple experience: I am connected deeply to everything else, and the wellbeing of the whole is my wellbeing also.

We are all aware of having connections, particularly with people in our families or people whom we like or with whom we work; we're all aware that we're dependent upon certain others to do things for us when we need them. When I need to travel, I may be dependent on the employees of the airline company—and particularly upon the pilots of the plane I'm in—to assure I and my baggage arrive safely at my destination. When I'm sick, I'm dependent on my doctor and perhaps on the staff in a hospital. For food, I'm dependent on my local grocer and on all the transportation people who get the food to his store and, of course, on the farmers and the natural world from which the food comes in the first place.

For a mystic, though, this sense of connectedness and mutual interdependency goes much deeper. The obvious links that make our everyday lives run smoothly are important, but there are unseen, less obvious connections that weave us all into a profound web of life. A mystic is someone who is sensitive to these deeper links, who is aware that there is more going on beneath the surface that ties us one to another in a dynamic system of constantly evolving wholeness.

The mystical life is one that is sensitive to the presence of wholeness and to its efforts to emerge in situations where it is not so apparent or has yet to manifest itself. Sometimes this sensitivity arises paradoxically from losing wholeness by being broken up and broken open.

This is what happened to Ruth, the author of this amazing book.

When she had her stroke and lost part of her brain function, as she describes, she became disconnected from her normal human world. The familiar threads of speech and words with which we ordinarily weave ourselves together with the world around us became lost to her. She had to discover new connections, new threads, new ways of weaving. She had to rediscover how to manifest the innate wholeness of her life and her connectedness with the rest of creation. She had to demonstrate that while we might break away from it for one reason or another, the world itself is never broken; it's unbrokenness remains for us to rediscover and reengage in new ways.

Which is exactly what mystics do. They are the artists of wholeness, the engineers of connectedness. And in particular, they are explorers of the connections we don't usually see, the wholeness that is not immediately apparent but which is there nonetheless under the surface.

When I first met Ruth, I knew I was in the presence of a remarkable person even before I heard the story of her stroke and her subsequent journey of healing. I viewed her as a true mystic even though she lives in no cloister and doesn't wear the trappings of a religious life. She is a brilliant psychotherapist and a most original artist, and through her work and life she demonstrates the wholeness-evoking love that is the hallmark of a true mystic.

It has been a privilege to know Ruth and to work with her. Now through her book, you are going to have that delight as well.

Preface

These are my stories losing language in a stroke, then brain trauma. I'm a clinical psychologist, psychoanalyst, baby observer, bird watcher. My sense of self survived using these skills to reflect on walking through a wilderness without road signs. I found languages outside of verbal language that took me to whole new worlds.

Oliver Sachs' piece in The New Yorker, "Recalled to Life" is the profound inspiration for this memoir. His piece took my breath away. He's a clinical neurologist telling an exquisite story of a woman who had totally lost expressive speech, told of her capacity to make a life anyway. As aphasic myself I marveled at his sensitivity to her life's condition. His was a really good story from the outside; I thought what if she could tell the story from the inside of such loss to complement his? A few weeks later I thought, maybe I can do this. So began the genesis of a five year journey to find language and memory to tell such a story of the inner experience.

To speak at all was to locate the fewest words to express anything. I wanted to keep this spare language to convey the unimaginable. Digging deep, then deeper again, I rooted into memory to illuminate for those who can't imagine the loss of language. And I wanted to speak for those thousands who have lost language and can't ever tell you how it is.

Between 2005 and 2008 an estimated 7 million people in the US had a stroke, nearly 800 thousand people -- on average every 40 seconds. 83% of those survive—most with some handicapping condition, 664 thousand people. The statistics for heart attacks are similar. Stroke, heart attack, cancer, and upper respiratory disease are the top four.

These events bring a person to death or within a hair's-breadth of dying, as I was.

To survive these moments of physical-spiritual choice between life and death is profound. It is also a choice point to make new life. From choosing cutting edge surgery to coping with loss of language, to making art, there was a long time to rethink, to recreate my life's meaning. Catastrophe comes with deep choices: One can fall apart emotionally, be miserable about the unfairness, or pick up the challenge and reenter life with vitality whatever the personal conditions.

These stories are about what it means to survive, what it means to find a place to live well despite circumstance.

Ruth Codier Resch, September 15, 2012

PART ONE:
THE PRECIPITOUS ABYSS

The heartbreaking collapse begins moments off an international Air Portugal jet in JFK airport. I'm returning with my research assistant from a successful presentation in Estoril, walking eagerly down the wide, busy hallway toward customs, international baggage, and home.

Suddenly,

my body folds in half; still standing on my feet... my eyes gaze inches from my toes.... why can't i hear? ... then i hear like through a fish tank. time suspends.

the bags that were on my shoulder are every-which-way across the floor.

What? ... i'm disoriented...then my hearing clears as i stand

something terrible. I'm vaguely terrified, nothing coheres. why are my bags are strewn about my feet?

i turn to my research assistant traveling with me . . .

but i can not speak! there are no words coming to my mouth! i can see the perfect mundane beige of the tiled floor. she talks. i listen but pay little attention. i am acutely terrified now. i have to tell her that. with no words, I struggle, "ca...... ...n't ... .sp...... ...ea.........k."

Her face fidgets around her eyes trying not to look alarmed. She says, lightly, "Maybe it is like ears clogging up with the descent of the plane and will resolve."

"N...o...o!" I say.

She chats about passport control, luggage, customs, anything to soften the charged air of desperation around me.

i am falling into a daze. i can't grasp what is happening ..... the breath in my chest is blurry, edgy ...i'm thinking ... but not in words ...

Donna takes charge. I wait for her in a the lounge area near the end of customs those rows of stuck-together chairs. She is somewhere behind the barrier, getting us both through baggage then customs. My body doesn't relax into the vinyl. I'm afraid, anxious for her to appear, wildly anxious. This isn't me. I've stepped into another me, some other universe, full of fear, veiled reality, steeped in ambiguity.

A tailored flight attendant stops in the corridor near me, notices my ashen, tense face, asks, "Are you OK?" I turn to her and shake my head. She tells me there is a medical center in the airport, maybe I want to check in there. I nod a thank-you, and she hurries on.

So quietly full of myself as I get off the jet. I've just presented my first paper using video, the new technology for baby research, to an international infant research conference in Portugal. I am forty-four. It is 1980. I'm just five years out from my clinical psychology doctorate. I pulled myself up from the depression of divorce, neither asked for, and took the opportunity to do the doctoral work I had wanted to do since I was sixteen.

My research is a mother-baby natural observation nursery. A group of mothers with their young babies comes and plays for the morning. I video; early emotion is the paper I gave in Portugal. I teach psychiatrists observation methods, supervise doctoral students, have a small private practice. Incredibly I am living my professional dream.

I have no idea as I sit waiting in a daze, the dream is gone.

Two days ago Donna and I went on a retreat after the conference into the lush, rugged mountains up behind Estoril. She went walking through the woods to find a long wooden stair down to a small lake. I stayed, sunning in the pension's small tree lined garden, relaxing on a long chaise. A terrible headache blasted into the peace. I was suddenly angry that she was gone so long, even that she went without me. Why so angry? I wondered, confused. It didn't really matter what she was doing. But the pain in my head kept pounding ... pounding… pounding…. mercilessly. I tried to nap, and hours later it went away. We had a fine dinner in the little pension, and the next day went to explore flea markets in Lisbon in the perfect sunshine before we taking the plane home.

Schlepping our bags now, we take a shuttle to the medical center, a small building in the center of the huge oval that is the many separate airline terminals of JFK.

In the hallway I argue wordlessly with the doctor, who refuses to let Donna in the examining room with me. There is a cold glitter in me as I grasp to her arm, agitated out of my mind. "Her! ... Me!" I point at her and then me, then us together. I manage the two pronouns, but I can't tell him anything else. I can't imagine why he doesn't want a talking person there with him. I won't know what to do with what he says. I must have her to speak for me and to hear. Under my pushy silence I am wild with fear.

He is clearly irritated. I'm insistent, lean into her, hold on. Finally he motions us to a small, bare room, an old wood desk like teachers used to have and a simple cot, no examining table. A cursory neurological exam. I've watched better in pediatric neurology clinic. Indifferent he says, "You've had a neurological event. Go home and call your doctor."

Just how would I do that, this going home and calling my doctor? I imagine walking into the office in my apartment. It is dark. I can barely see my wide teak desk in the gloom, or the phone on top of the answering machine sitting on the far corner. I wonder where my doctor's number is. For that matter, what is my doctor's name?

I imagine dialing a number and getting it wrong over and over ... and over. Suppose I do manage to dial, and I hear a voice at the end of line.

"Doctor's office."

THEN WHAT? Sitting in examining room, I burst into tears. What could I say . . .

without words?

Donna and the doctor have left. On the cot, I huddle into myself, alone, more and more frantic. A nurse comes in, "Why are you crying!" Her voice is curt, unkind. I want say, "The doctor hasn't told me anything about my condition. 'Neurological event' isn't specific, and he has given me a plan I can't do." Fear and anger try to meld, but I can't speak to the awful frustration inside.

My thoughts are clear and bright. I think that they are words, but they roll like video pictures. It is an altered reality, badly done, corrupt. I cry helplessly. It is hopeless in this room. I wipe the tears and snot on my sleeve and follow the nurse out.

Donna is in the reception area, filling out paper work, looks at me with a nod. Dread compels me to my address book somewhere in my bags near her. I find it and struggle to think of my doctor's name. R pops up. I thumb to the R's. Ha! There is his name! She calls, is given instructions for the hospital to take me to.

It is late March. Rush hour, a monsoon rain and a subway strike. An ambulance isn't more efficient than a taxi they tell us, so we opt for the cab, not thinking at all that I might need medical oversight. The rain on the Long Island Expressway is heavy and pounding; the brilliance of the highway lights is reflected in the wet roadway. The taxi's familiar Naugahyde scent feels warm, cozy. The friendly driver, the sound of the rain is calming. I will be in a hospital soon. My doctor waiting.

But I am not calm. The fiasco in the medical center, the useless information, have unhinged me. I can't think what medical problem would just take away my speech, poof! while I remain walking around, schlepping my bags, and able get into this nighttime cab. Other thoughts begin to plague me. Will they think it's psychological because I can't tell them anything? What if they get it wrong like One Flew over the Cuckoo's Nest and I'm stuck in some terrible box forever? Fear infuses everything, even the warm cab, the rainy night, scorching, heavy, like a storm I can't see beyond.

In the Emergency Room, Donna straggling my bags behind me, I stammer my name, "Dddooocteer Ruuutttth...." She stops me, "We're expecting you." My body floods with relief. I follow limply where she tells me. The unknown is draped everywhere in front of me like a dense brocade curtain, confusing and obscuring.

A blur of residents examines me for hours, first in the ER then after I'm admitted, ask questions I can't answer. I know what they want, but can't say. I've changed the time on my watch during the flight to New York time, but my body is on Portugal time. I can't tell them it is five in the morning; I'm desperate to sleep. Two of them now talk among themselves urgently. I know they are working hard to give a report to my doctor in the morning. But I feel like a fish flopping on the concrete.

I'm clearer the next day when my doctor visits. He asks, "Was there anything else medical that happened in Portugal?" Yes, yes, I must aid in his diagnostic puzzle ...

For the whole day I struggle to find the words. I search... two words to answer ... find them ...lose them... search again, find ... only to lose again. Practice, practice, to remember.

Finally when he comes, I speak the two words to him, point to my armpit.

"in...fe...cti..on.... an..ti..bio...tic!"

He orders a spinal tap for infection and finds it clear.

I have a neurologist now. I see him bustle down the hall, his fitted white coat over modish suit, his residents running fast behind him. They all burst through the door, then stay clustered there like huddled jocks waiting for the signals for the rush to play. The neurologist, tall and quite handsome, is doing teaching rounds with them. I see them in a far distance as if I'm looking through a tube. They stay at the door, don't come near me, speak to me, or examine me. Still, I feel a like a specimen.

From the podium of the chart, he explains my case to them. He announces to the room, "She has expressive aphasia." I know this already, not the word aphasia, but the loss of words. Then he says, "She has comprehension intact!" Yes, yes, this is true! I DO understand everything I hear from them:

doctors, nurses, the close friends that come! Yes, thank you. I have a mind that understands. Thank you, thank you!

I want to gesture gratitude, but my hands just lie there on the white sheets. They aren't paralyzed, they simply don't move to mime thought. Inert. Like my mind, they have also lost expression.

I had plans to be in Connecticut soon to present the same paper to a child development conference. I want the doctors to finish this up and release me. I've a life to get on with.

Days later I tell my doctor, "Lea…ve . . . pa…per," and gesture getting out of bed. He says nothing. No reality checks, no soothing argument, no "I'm sorry, you can't leave." The nothing he says resounds.

In shock, I haven't seen the enormity of what has happened to my life. It is a shambles at my feet, a disaster. I could just give up … let go of life, face being nothing, a vegetable…. but I'm alive!….it's a muddle.

Then a few days later I find a few words more, some seem possible. But I don't see the now of what is wrong with me, so I can't see a future. My life is in limbo.

I think of my internship. The neuropsychologist said, "Positive change in function bodes well in cases of brain damage." Good, this is change.

I imagine a black box, words locked inside, no door, only a few words drifting outside. Wordless thoughts come … and go. . Still, I can't see a future apart from this white place. My life is in limbo.

I'm taken to many tests and scans across many days: cat scan, some kind of nuclear body scan as if I'm in a metal sandwich, a cerebral angiogram, x-rays, blood studies. Each time the tech says my name, reassures me I'm known.

Finally my doctor says, "You've had a stroke, but we don't know why … yet. You are young for this."

"Ohh….hh….fu…c…k!" It is not a word; it is an outburst, an expletive. Now I do feel the enormity of what he's told me, but that, too, is locked in the black box. There is so little to express my thoughts, my questions to him.

"We'll continue to look and see what can be done for you," he says.

"Is she always like this, so placid?" the neurologist asks my friend Kathy, a neuropsychologist, a few days after the stroke.

"No, definitely not!"

I have little urgency, that's true. I'm not railing with frustration, no active angst. Placid is the right word. This is not me.

Mornings later I think: Time to have a good cry. I've tucked the crisp sheets and white spread around my shoulders. I feel safe here in this room; nurses are kind, change my room when I can't sleep because of the putrid smell of my roommate's continuous enema, put "Quiet" signs on my door. The doctors are carefully informative as they get more results from tests. But as I look out into the empty white corridor, my life is broken; I am, myself, unsafe.

I want to be angry, want big feelings to well up into my eyes. Tears don't come to swell emotion into form. They, too, are locked inside. I'm a crier; this is unnerving. I let it go and wait.

Another day. Nothing, no tears. I'm frightened this time; reflect without words, this is radically wrong. I think this, but only distantly. Expressing emotion—my very selfness—is locked in the box along with the words. I can't bear to notice I'm not myself. I put the thought away in a roadless wilderness.

Close friends make a fortress of protective secrecy around me knowing I'm fragile without words. Even in my crusty independence they know I wouldn't know now how to say, Enough!

Jake comes every couple of days, folds herself sideways into a chair at the bottom of my bed, legs over the arm, and regales me with stories of her journey to see me. I'm captured by her eccentric word pictures. She meets old friends on the street in our neighborhood; she knows everyone.

Clothing attracts her eye this day, the dash of a patterned scarf, the chic line of a suit, the causal saunter of the wearer. She is visual with words. She describes the personalities of the dogs she sees, the black lab puppy that seems to giggle with her body in happiness when Jake leans down to talk to her. A golden retriever holds his head high as if he doesn't notice her admiration. She laughs at his hauteur.

I see in her words the soft quality of the clear day as she rounds the corner from Pierrepont Street into Henry toward the subway. I see pictures of her world that I don't have to copy into words. It is a movie, gives me very sweet pleasure, entertains me, no effort, cheering.

Only my closest friends get to visit me. Two colleagues get through the fortress anyway, bustle in with high energy. They haven't come together. They are especially delighted to see each other and arrange themselves to either side of my bed. I don't expect these particular two. I'm abashed. But I slowly put together a few words for them, extremely slowly. "Pl..ea...se ...slow....dow..n..." They don't wait to give me time, don't listen while I struggle. They begin to talk vibrantly to each other across my body. I might as well not be here. But I AM here.

That they ignore me hurts, and their loud, fast talk above me hurts my brain more. I'm lost in their high energy, can't summon a word to tell them, to protect myself. I'm overwhelmed in physical misery. I wait them out ... till they go.

This is chaos – of mind, of spirit. I've fallen into this abyss without warning, healthy, young, and now invisible.

A hospital volunteer comes by with a small cart of books from the patient library. I don't know how to tell her a preference, so she suggests a mystery. Every few days she brings me a slim Simenon French mystery or a fat LeCarré MI5 British spy story. They entertain my bland hours between the excitements of going for tests and crucial visits of doctors giving results and explanations. The doctors give me no certainties.

The books are tangible, solid. But the stories I read come in and go out of my head. I don't recall what I have read; there are no words to make a summary in my mind. There is the present moment of reading, and then it is gone.

I wait for the other stories the doctors may tell me about my brain.

I've been in the hospital for a month, and the doctors discharge me with a pill to take once a day for blood thinning. Kathy is definitive, not happy with this treatment plan. She jeers, "Tiny orange pill!" I take the doctor's word. I'm happy to be home, reattaching to the bigger world. But Kathy is right—the little pill doesn't hold the onslaught. In a bare two weeks I'm re-hospitalized, mini-strokes, TIAs. I'm put on serious IV blood thinners. In the quiet of the hospital I can feel them softly hurry across my brain.

It is unstable; I know I can have another big one.

I tell nurses whenever the little mini-strokes happen. One reassures me, "Perhaps it's anxiety."

"No! ….not ….li…ke… th…at!" I exclaim hotly to her brush-off. I try not to be terrified. One Flew Over the Cuckoo's Nest runs through my mind again. My life is too close to the edge.

The various films don't look like anything the doctors have seen before. They have no treatment, only the IV blood thinners. They present my case to clinical case conferences in all the major hospitals in the city. I am the mystery case.

The hospital has a little rooftop garden. It is early summer, and I'm allowed to take my IV pole down the elevator. I shed my hospital gown and for awhile soak in the sun wearing a trumped-up bright blue bikini from my underwear, dreaming I'm on the sand at Fire Island. Visitors come, admire my growing tan. Then a nurse calls from a high window that doctors want me, and the dream beach shatters.

This story is broken, like my language. Before and after are mixed up, like my speech, little sequences, shards. I can't convey how it is inside this crucible as though it's a regular narrative. It's not lived that way. Later maybe, but not now.

I'm stepping outside to reflect. The inside self and the thoughts are lost from connection to others. I'm in existential shock, living in the moment. It is a practical matter, not enlightenment. Ordinary life is gone.

The narrative, like my words, is disordered … patchy … shards … fragment moments, like broken sentences. My mind is not a deranged or idiot mind, but a mind trying slowly to see itself, to articulate without steady expression. There isn't a road in front of me, no visible signposts to guide. Without words, signposts, and markers of forks and intersections, the path itself is gone.

Not just that my life is irrevocably changed, but the essence of my very being is being altered. Life, reduced to crushing small pieces of moment, is losing the foundation, the arc of personal narrative. Small events are the dramatic tension. Single events placed side by side, by side, by side, like single words on a charm bracelet.

I pick up the shards as though there were a narrative, as though the path I knew, or any path, were visible. That is what I'm doing. Brave, valiant, necessary, but not real. I don't know how to invent a life. I use the pieces that are still left lying around. They are the only narrative there is, small events.

Any stroke is unique; they are like that, each one physiologically different. One recovers or dies. But the loss of language is not unique. One lives with it in its many forms. At least a quarter of a million people each year in this country alone fall newly into this wilderness of aphasia through stroke, brain injury, or disease. I can barely articulate what is happening. I experience no storyline, little past, no future in my mind. Not memory loss. I am flooded by the present—one word at a time.

Without words to organize and plan my mind's intentions, there is only my vibrating body, at a loss, at sea, thundering waves. I'm not used to living in my body; I'm in pre-school with this. That is the crux of it. My mind works, but in tatters.

I'm telling inner experience here, wrenching it out of liminal mind, sensory memory, sometimes out of shear nervy intestine. It is the outside view that provides a narrative, a meaning. Inside here, where it is lived, there isn't a trajectory of words, or the possibility for it. Daily bravery, loss, perseverance, falling apart aren't a narrative by themselves.

It is the death card. Clear. On the table. It permeates everything. I'm discharged for the afternoon from one hospital to another for a neurosurgical consult. I am eager to be out in the world, being caged for two months now — with only the scant two weeks home. I want to taste life out there, behind these walls.

I imagine the sweetness of sitting with my daughter and Jake in a cozy little French restaurant somewhere on the Upper West Side, looking at supper menus, after the consultation. The discharge nurse seems to listen in on my thoughts of escape and tells me severely, "You can't go anywhere else, only come back here!" For that moment, elegant dining together, I wanted the pretense of being normal, in the world.

When I do step into the street for a taxi, I am assailed by the clamor, the sounds, the commotion of people. I'm giddy, feel faint … unshielded.

Carefully planning, we are on time, but the doctor is not. We wait on big brown leather couches in the reception room of Neurological Institute, part of Presbyterian Hospital. I am wearing real clothes and wait like an ordinary person. The illusion is thin, and I begin to suffer. I wonder: Don't they realize I'm a hospital patient? No one is watching over me here. I wish I were in hospital clothes and had come in an ambulance. The energy I had is seeping away — crowds in the street, the rushing taxi, the excitement of being outside, the anticipation of the consultation. My body feels frail and frantic … this waiting. An hour has gone by. Fear is clothed in flagging energy. I am unsafe.

I think of asking Jake to complain for me, but I can't summon the words for the deeper sense of catastrophe in my body. I wait. Nothing shows on the outside.

At last Dr. James Correll, the neurosurgeon, brings us into his examining room. He had been studying my angiogram x-rays before we came in and now puts them up on his light box for us to see.

My daughter and Jake, a veteran of many surgeries, are my Board of

Directors for this. I had prodded them beforehand to ask many questions, even the ones that seem too simple. "Ask … dumb … ques … tions," I pleaded, my speech being a little better. I must have them be auxiliary mind and memory for me, to hear and think for me, as Donna did at the airport medical center. I'm slow to process information into my own words and thoughts. I'm prepared for things to go too fast.

My other doctors make pencil diagrams for me and don't let me see the actual x-rays. And here they are in front of me. A reality.

A brief neurological exam, then Dr. Correll takes us through the x-rays methodically, explaining carefully to us what he sees in each image.

"There is a clot wedged into the wall of the artery here," he says. He bends toward the x-ray, tracing the four major arteries with his finger, and then points to the left interior one.

"Here! It's too far up in the artery to try to pull out … and it is wedged in."

I lean over and peer at the film where he points and see only a blob in the murk. This has been the center of mystery and discussion among my doctors and the many others they presented to around the city. Dr. Correll's name came up as the one to consult.

His voice is gentle. He speaks slowly, leaving me time for thought, and with language that is clear and precise.

Then he explains how he would use very new microsurgery technology to cut out the whole artery with the clot in it, a very new procedure for the brain. He points to the interior artery where the cut would be made. My body strains forward toward the picture, hoping to comprehend better what he shows me.

"Then," he says, "we will take one of the branches of the left exterior artery, here … the one that goes around the side of your face," tracing it on the angiogram. "We will place it into the damaged speech area of your brain. The branch, in time, will grow into a whole new blood supply for you!"

I struggle against fuzzing out and letting my daughter and Jake think for me … against the overwhelm of words, the complexity and the hugeness of what he is suggesting.

He waits and he waits for me, going through it again and again, waiting until we all understood enough of it, responding to our many questions.

He takes us to his adjacent his office to sit with me. He knows I am a clinical psychologist, and honors the mind behind the flagging speech. He goes through the differential diagnosis for the condition he sees. He explains that there are four possibilities for causing the dissecting aneurysm he has diagnosed. He easily rules out three of them, and I agree as he speaks. The last is an accident in the last five days before the stroke. "No recent accident," I tell him. "but," very slowly I explain, "ten years ago I slipped …. fell straight down…. on my butt …. unconscious briefly….. taken to the ER….. eventually diagnosed with a brain concussion, no testing."

I remember the day. George and I had sold our three-quarters renovated house on the edge of Brooklyn Heights and bought a magnificent 1880's mansion at a low price on the edge of Park Slope just off Flatbush. Almost pristine; we were the third owners. I was walking with two cups of coffee from the tiny modern kitchen with its amber and green stained-glass window through the dining room toward the room with the second-story turret with a spire rising into the sky. The floors had been finished with the new polyurethane, but I'd waxed them anyway. Quite suddenly my feet slipped beneath me, and I refused to let go of the cups. I fell straight down on my tush with a hard crash. I got up, went back to the kitchen intending … what? A cloth to wipe up the spills? Get more coffee? I became dizzy, and fainted. George called 911.

A few months later George and I parted. I call the beautiful old house my castle in the air.

The clot being discussed now is directly above the top of my spine. When I fell, my spine smashed into my brain. It has taken all this time to cause trouble. The neurosurgeon turns to speak about surgery, leans slightly across the large, old, dark mahogany desk toward me.

"We would like to do this for you."

There isn't a medical polish to the words, only an ease and simplicity that softens in my body. I feel like he is extending an elegant coat for me to consider. I'm soothed by this kind gesture. I feel his patience as a form of precision that makes my body feel calm and clear. I am in the presence of a master. I feel it in my bones—I am willing to put my life in his hands.

He is one of five neurosurgeons in the world who can do this surgery. It is that new. He tells me I would be his seventh patient, and it would be a long surgery, ten or twelve hours.

My life is on the line in this room.

He disappears, inaccessible to my doctors for three days. I am impatient for them to get on with it, to find out whatever we need to know. They examine and question me incessantly, trying to understand the story I've given them. I tell and retell as best as I can. They are in a huddle, like basketball players, going over and over the team strategies for the possible plays. The story I've given them is totally new, and they are surprised by it. They want a report from the surgeon to understand the reasoning for both the diagnosis and such a radical surgery. They, too, are impatient; for the moment they have only me.

I watch Dr. Correll come down the long, dark mahogany paneled hall of this magnificent old hospital. The little milky sconces tucked along the wall cast an edgy glimmer around the crisp white of his lab coat. There is something odd about his walk, I think; his coming in the afternoon to see me can't be good.

"Here's my doctor!" I tell the assembly, my close friends and my mother. They've come together here in the solarium, a send-off party for my brain surgery tomorrow morning. The high, thick windows send bright gray light into the room. The presence of my friends and their gaiety softens the solitary loneliness of tomorrow. I might not see them again.

"He's low to the ground!" two of my medical friends standing against the wall exclaim at the same time. I frown at them.

Wise cracking, I think.

"No," one explains getting my thought, "he will have better endurance for standing for a long surgery … this is a good thing!"

The neurosurgeon, indeed a short man, comes into the room, looks around, smiling at the convivial crowd. We are sipping fine brandy from plastic glasses. He sits down at a table beside my mother, but his face turns serious.

"We've been bumped again!" he says to the room at large.

The room tenses around me, but it's my heart that has fallen to the floor. I've been admitted to this hospital for this surgery, and this is the second time it has been postponed in the OR schedule. The first time a gunshot wound to the head in a street fight took priority … over my fragile brain.

"The surgery will not be tomorrow, but Friday for sure!" His voice is emphatic. He doesn't tell me why this time.

My mother's voice rises into the taut stillness, edged with a shrill. She leans toward him, her small, square frame defiant. "But that's Friday the thirteenth! We can't have that!" Her voice hits me like a stun gun; my body goes numb, my skin hot with irritation.

What WE does she speak for? Is she walking in my shoes?

She has been quiet today, but for the last few days she has been raging at my friends. I asked them to look after her, but they can't get near her sizzling armor. Not even Kathy, my toughest friend.

I swallow my feelings and slowly search for words. I cannot touch her intensity. Behind her rage are hidden tendrils of love; she is desperate to stave off the specter of my death. She rushes headlong to embrace this superstition she doesn't believe.

My fear is specific. With a sudden, bigger stroke, my mind could become a vegetable before they get me into the OR. If that happens, death is preferable.

I lean around my mother to face the surgeon. I say quietly to him, "I'm … ready … when … you are!

The morning of Friday the thirteenth finally comes. My body sinks into a lush comforter of calm; my fear has left the building. The light coming in the window of my small room is blue-gray and soft this morning. My mood, too, is soft and expectant. My mother and a patient from across the hall come, sit quietly with me. When the nurse comes with the corsage of sedations and bundles me up in warm blankets, I'm ready to put on the beautiful coat the surgeon seemed to offer to me in his office. I slip onto the gurney.

The doors to the OR suite are old shining oak with large windows, and swing out to welcome me in. The neurosurgeon is standing there, dapper in street clothes and white lab coat. He receives me, a graceful moment. Pulling my coat more tightly about me, I am satisfied. He turns half away from me, commanding the OR staff behind him, "OK folks, let's get moving! We have a lot of work to do!" Then motions the transport to take me to a tiny anesthesia cubby down the hall.

Once under anesthesia my inert body is ushered into an ultra-hi-tech surgery. The neurosurgeon works on my brain through a large microscope. His chief nurse monitors through another eyepiece to watch and anticipate the instruments he will want. The anesthesiologist explained to me yesterday the left side of my head will be shaved and a wide crescent shape in my skull will be very carefully sawed open. This is the first part of the surgery: the surgeon selects one of the branches of the exterior artery and places it into the expressive speech area to give a new blood supply. Its many tiny branch ends are stapled shut in their new places. When the first part is stable and secure, the second part is done: an incision is made in my neck, and the artery with the clot in it is cut and the whole length of it in my brain is pulled away.

Many nurses, residents, and neurosurgery fellows rotate in and out to do support work and to learn. A medical friend gets reports from them as they come out. If the surgery should go badly, he has my instructions for the surgeon. Let me die peacefully.

After eight long hours, I'm sedated semi-conscious in the ICU for three days, tucked inside the elegant coat. Residents rouse me, prick my feet with a pin, shine a light in first one eye and then the other, and ask me to repeat, Methodist Episcopal. I fall back asleep, and they leave, come back, over and over again.

I'm blurry, beginning to waken, disconnected, still in and out of sleep. The first person I see is my analyst. I haven't seen her in ten years. Seeing her, I know that I am OK. I have survived.

I'm suddenly fragile standing here. My new rearranged brain is slow to take in this little world of quiet side street, but I am softly exultant. I am stepping into my life again. I am alive!

I've been in two hospitals for most of three months, held in a cocoon. The narrative of my life held in the wrap. This one is an old brick building standing quietly and grandly on a dead-end side street. I have pushed ahead to step into the delicate sun, eager to taste the day. Jake, behind me, is managing my stuff, my bags, my flotsam. Released from the door, I gasp in pleasure. Alone in this quiet street, I feel a green and silver newness. Today it is all over, the cocoon ripped open. I am going home.

Here in the street my life shreds a little: a patch of now… another patch of now… shards. I'm mortal now. I've seen my death, and it walks with me. Out here in the street, I know it in my body, my remade brain. I've survived. I can only think of being home.

Jake tells the taxi driver to drive down the West Side through Riverside Park rather than take the highway. I turn outward to the world to drink the sunshiny trees, dogs barking, the twinkly hues of the gray Hudson River. Familiar sights of the city come into view, high-rises, warehouses, the Marina, the Battery, Brooklyn Bridge. They are all awesome to me, one by one. Then the vast energy of everything around me comes up from the ground, hurls itself into the taxi, and pummels my body. Suddenly this world is too much.

I expect a haven when I walk into my Brooklyn Heights apartment. Instead an awkward unfamiliarity assails me. It isn't the home I left, flying off to Portugal months ago. My comfortable living room with its velvety blue and green striped couch, the soft brown loveseat, and the Oriental red and blue narrow runner down the center: they don't reach out to envelop me. My eyes pop out the big windows to the view across the Brooklyn rooftops toward the immensity of lower Manhattan. It is all too bright.

I am dazed, a stranger in my own apartment. I stand for a time, search for the ordinary familiarity of the place. Jake and my daughter fuss around me, to welcome me, help me settle. My skin is irritable. My eyes and my skin draw into themselves against the bright largeness. I wish I were wrapped once more in the cocoon. I retreat to my room, the polished teak desk, the leather chairs. The light is dim and restful. I put my body gingerly onto the bed. I'm happy to be here, but my brain is battered, clanging with all the sensations of coming home.

The telephone rings and rings, too much sound, too much sensation. My jumbled brain boils over the top and turns painful. I feel no rest in my prone body. I beg Jake and my daughter, "Please, please … I can't … can't talk … to anyone…. too much." I want to see and talk to friends, but I'm raw. My body here at home is out of time, out of place. I am not normal; I have to begin living in this skin.

The next day I crave to be outside. I walk with one of my friends the short blocks down Pierrepont to the Promenade overlooking Manhattan, leisurely and slowly. I am content in my neighborhood, thirsty for its sights.

My eyes stroll the nineteenth-century details of the Greek revival townhouses, the curling celery leaves fashioned inside scrolls of stone. Some are reddish brownstone, others white limestone. Their variety decorates my walk, and my eyes follow the lines of black wrought iron railings individually cast for each house a century ago.

It is high summer and window boxes bloom with color, cared for by people behind tall windows. I cannot express to my keeper how deeply good it is to be out in the world again, the grace of my ordinary neighborhood. I gulp in visual detail with the tenderness of loss and return.

My breath heaves in my chest, and I'm compelled to stop. I have been walking only the short halls of medical wards. As we approach the Promenade, the towering buildings of Manhattan across the East River are too vast, too overwhelming. I shrink from the magnificent walk I wanted. Instead we stop in the little toddler playground next to the Promenade. Trees and bushes circle it. I'm enclosed in green.

Toddlers giggle and shriek as they move gray and brown sand with yellow shovels into red and blue buckets. They lean against the little concrete wall or climb up it, thinking carefully about where to put each hand, boost a knee up to hands and then to stand on top. Scampering across the walk, they throw themselves, laughing, into a mother's lap.

I long for the sweetness of the babies and mothers in my research nursery. A light breeze ruffles my hair. It was combed over my half-shaved head and now my naked scalp opens to the air. I laugh, as it feels good in the breeze, but I push the hair around again to cover it so the long arc of raw incision doesn't shock. It's good here in this little grove, and I'm happy watching the toddlers. Out of the hospital, life feels precious in its exquisite details.

My stamina fades and we start back. I feel the hot pressure of the sun, and my body crumples onto nearby steps. I rest a moment, thinking to get up, but the expansiveness I felt in the playground is gone. "Let's get a taxi!" my friend says. It feels like a silly thing to do for three blocks, but when it arrives, my grateful body crawls into its sanctuary.

In the middle of the night I wake with terrible cramps in my legs. I need to go to the bathroom, but my legs won't move me out of bed. I call out to my daughter, asleep in her room on the other side of the kitchen. I try to shout again and again.

Part of the surgery was close to my voice box, and it is bruised. My shout is a pathetic whisper. She will never hear this. I am getting desperate for the bathroom.

The telephone on the floor is a solution. I dial the phone in her room and get a sleepy voice.

"I'm sor...ry to wak...e you li...ke this," I say, "I can't... ge...t ...out ... of ...bed."

She mumbles with an irritated edge. She is not awake.

"I NE...ED ...TO G...O ....TO TH...E... BA....THRO...OM... AND I.... CA..N'T GE...T UP!"

"Oh!" she says. "OK."

I am afraid she may go back to sleep, but a moment later I hear her shuffling feet, and she appears in the doorway. Her face grimaces with the sudden light in my room.

Sheepish this time, I say, "I cann...'t... get... up. I have... to go... real bad." She is gentle as she helps me up. I have slept naked for the hot night and try to pull the sheet modestly around me. In hopping to the bathroom, it falls away. She holds her arms around me, lifting me strongly. I am sobbing as I sink onto the toilet. "There, there," she says softly, "it's OK now." I feel like a naked baby and a demented old lady.

She massages my legs and gets us glasses of iced tea. There is no going back to sleep, so she stretches out on my bed and rests her back against the wall. She tells me how things have been for her in the last months at school since I got sick and what she was thinking about her courses next fall and her current boyfriend. I am mostly listening; my helplessness has made us open to one another. It is good to hear her talk about her life. In the sweetness of this intimacy, it doesn't matter that I speak sparely.

The night is long. No pressure.

I imagine myself in my baby observation research nursery resuming work. I want to do this. I see the mothers and the babies, the video cameras, the smart research assistant, the psychiatry residents observing in canvas director's chairs around the edges of the mock living room I set up. The mothers have come for the morning and chat together on couches as they too watch their babies. They play on the large blue green nubbly rug, crawling and squealing to their mothers, mouthing and exploring toys. They play parallel to one another, but nonetheless they are social in this. There is a video console in a corner where I watch three screens from different cameras in the room. I record the ordinary little separations between baby and mother. It is a sweet vision. I can't imagine how I can restart it all.

I try to write a note to one of my students who sent me flowers in the hospital when he wasn't supposed to know where I was. I want to write, "What a wonderful surprise…" to start and then chide him for getting through the fortress. I can't connect sound to letter to the word in my mind. "What letter is the wha sound or what letter is the th sound?" I ask myself, but I can't think what the letters that go with them. It's an automatic little task! I'm shocked and frightened, but still I can't sink into feeling. I can't even send the mothers notes about what has happened to me or why we won't continue in the fall.

I can't manage my checkbook. Another shock when the bank manager calls to alert me that my account is terribly overdrawn. I thought my adding and subtracting were fine. In the hospital I asked friends to fix my checkbook, but they wouldn't, none of them, too intimate. They would sooner wash out my underwear.

I can't conceive how to do the nursery, get it organized again, all the words. My god, all the words! It is painful to imagine I won't be able to do it again, the grant writing to keep it going, reconnecting with the mothers.

My daughter and I go on vacation a month or so after being home—a couple of weeks to a small island I love off the coast of Maine. Jake comes along.

My first time there was my honeymoon, a young twenty-one. George and I hitchhiked up from New York and stayed at the Trailing Yew, an old seacoast cottage with close-by buildings and bedrooms sparely furnished. There were communal, simple meals for the guests and genial talk among us all. He and I walked the headlands and the woods where children hid cunning fairy houses made from moss, pine needles, and pennies. We met no one on the trails and soaked up the peacefulness in our new love.

When our daughter was four or five, we took every August in the tiny aerie of the second floor, of the house called Uncle Henry's, that stood halfway up the cliff from the dock. The porch looked out across the ocean to the sunsets and the magnificence of the fog rolling in and out along the water. George, a calligrapher, book designer, and art photographer, spent his time along the high promontories on the far side of the island and along rocky edges of the water with his camera. I saw what he saw, heard what he was thinking. I tried out one of his cameras, but realized I had no vision for seeing through it. I saw that I would be a poor mimic of his seeing.

Tentatively I started to draw weeds, the little grasses and small puffballs on stems in the box on the porch railing. George showed me how bold strokes would catch the flair of the grasses better than my feathery strokes climbing up the stem. I drew weeds and wildflowers in the unmown yard

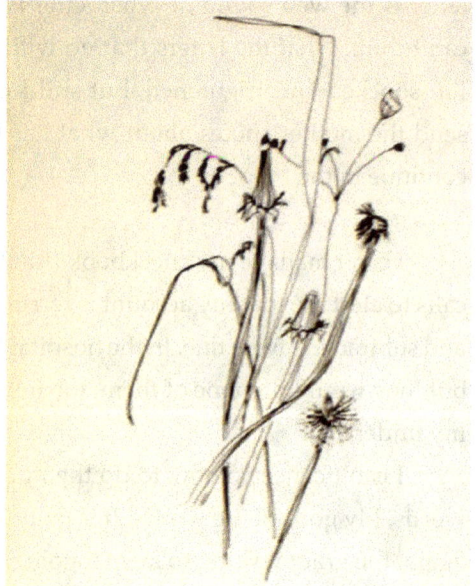

and then in the woods, always looking at the gestures and the patterns.

George would go back to the city in the middle of the month, and I learned to be alone with myself … and to draw.

I am eager now to walk with Jake and my daughter, eager for the remembered peacefulness of Cathedral Woods. Immensely tall and soaring pines make soft swishing sounds by light breezes in their tops. At their base the deep mulch of the seasons of needles spread a leathery brown covering, large and intimate at the same time. I am eager for the scrubby path and the scramble down to Pebble Beach where the "pebbles" are glacial boulders.

Walking with Jake, these visions in my head, my body gives out. I haven't the stamina. I want to go to the densely quiet woods in the center of the island and then out to the magnificent headlands on the other side. Too weak, I walk the little dirt road in the small village. I sit on the rocks near my room, watch the tide roll the kelp.

Even this quiet island world is too dazzling. A walk to the country store, seeing people I know along the way, is more than I can take. My fragile body churns with unmanageable sensation. The inside and outside sensations boil into a physical commotion that cascades into flood, like a baby being tickled into screaming, physical overload.

It used to be so simple to make words and have feelings at the same time. My halting words now are too gossamer to shelter the mass of sensation and emotion underneath the enduring calamities of my day. I haven't enough words to smooth all the jumbled pieces together. I'm trying valiantly to be in the world, but I'm unmoored. Behind my presence, ragged as it is, I know I'm coherent, sentient, even with the lack of words. Still … I'm not quite sure.

I have to retreat.

I borrow an ancient manual typewriter from the inn where we are staying. The inn stands at the top of the cliff, with a magnificent view of the ocean and the little islands close by. My room back down the hill is small, has no view, a little closed-in cocoon. I trudge down the hill with the typewriter and make a desk of a little table in the room.

Since I don't recognize sounds as letters, I cannot spell. I type fast to avoid thinking about spelling. I let my fingers use motor memory through another part of my brain. I am a terrible typist, and the result is pretty bad. I keep on anyway; it is good enough to see what I want to know.

Can my mind still articulate concepts? It is ... essential ... to know this. The paper I have in mind is based on videos in my research nursery of an autistic baby and her mother, their immense difficulty to form a sensory relationship. I write bits ... parts of ideas ... search. I cut with scissors, rearrange words, paste with glue. My pages are full of pasted pieces. I'm up early in the morning, typing, pushing for thought. The neighbor upstairs complains. I have only two more days.

I must get into the black box of words.

Two close friends, physicians, on their way to a shoreline walk, stop to chat as I'm sitting in an old rocking chair on the porch of my little room. When I tell them, slowly, that I am writing a paper, they stare off into space, faces blank, as though I hadn't spoken. What can they say?

Is it crazy even to think of writing a paper?

When I leave the island I'm triumphant. I have a few messy pasty pages. They are a start. Back in the city a colleague joins me in this endeavor, willing and very patient. Working in his office, I continue to stumble around, slowly writing, sorting words and ideas with him. We pass very rough drafts back and forth.

I'm knocking on the door of my verbal world. I am passionate for this, fiercely grasping shards from the shambles of my career.

Out in my neighborhood I struggle to speak in the halting, tattered grammar of a toddler. I have lost the ease of basic housekeeping speech: chit-chat, requests, questions.

The world's words rush past me. I hear, and there is no space for me to collect my thoughts or respond. The world outside is too fast for me to conjure the words. Time in my word mind is slow. Others forget I'm here.

Each time I speak I have to invent words anew. The stress and fatigue of it make the words I want fly away. When I make a request to the Korean green grocer around the corner, my words turn around themselves ... wrong sequence ... missed words ... "Pound...half... ...that!" I say "tomorrow" instead of "yesterday."

My life is narrowed to the moment, finding a word, another word, then another to try for a sentence. I lose the thread of the few words I've collected together in search for the next word. My body strains, holding all that effort of brain. It is not visible to others how hard it is.

It is early September. New York psychoanalysts return to their practices. Lemming-like, I do too. What is left for me is only my small private practice. I call two patients to resume work. All of the eight or so patients have been waiting for me these seven months, some waiting with other therapists. I am moved by their constancy.

I am naïve about continuing a practice, since no one has told me I can't. The only advice I've gotten is from a doctor after the surgery who said, "You are a high level aphasic; you don't need speech therapy. Just don't lift pianos."

My ability to listen and to speak just a few words should serve well enough. It doesn't. In session I hear what the patient says and understand the depth of it. I receive language, think about it. I think without words to think in. It is all in there, reflecting, observing, considering, comparing. But this observing mind doesn't translate into articulate organizing words for my verbal mind. What I think is far too complex for the slow small range of words I have for thinking.

I have a wordless mind trying to talk to a word mind. My thinking is a puzzle. I must find the pieces of words to construct a picture of my inner conversation. But most of the pieces are still in the black box. I clutch at the door, wrestle to pry it open, put my foot on the sill as a wedge, reach in, and scramble around to find pieces to fit. The struggle goes on even when I say nothing.

The practice is exhausting, but I continue. The work with patients is a deep pleasure to me. It is what is left to me of my professional identity—and my sole income now. In session I'm attentive and quietly elated. It is after the session when the fatigue slides in. Listening is my strength, inward and outward. I hear the emotions and thoughts patients express and feel empathy. My own emotions, though, don't rise to the surface as they did before. They don't clutter the emotional pathways between us. The practice has a certain simplicity in that way.

My daughter returns to college after the summer of taking care of me. She looks forward to classes, friends, fun, and study, but it doesn't happen. First, her father's mother dies, and then two weeks later her advisor dies suddenly while recuperating from a successful surgery. She tries to cope, but this is too much death in her face. She arranges a leave of absence for the semester and comes home.

It's no better at home for her; I am an unspoken, living face of death. Though I've escaped, I am deeply damaged. Home is not a relief. She becomes dramatic, angry, and emotional. I can't meet her emotions, her grief, with any expression of my own. I haven't the words to speak into the awful abyss of death. In the tumult she makes a plan and goes to stay with her father on the West Coast, giving herself a softer place of refuge.

A colleague invites me for a serene weekend to his home high on a cliff on the North Shore of Long Island. We walk the long stairs bounded by trees and bushes clinging to the fragile cliff to sit and talk on the fortified beach. He and his wife are interesting people, give me time to find words, talk seems easy. I enjoy the luxury of the quiet with them, away from the city.

Months later his wife tells me they thought me depressed, speaking so slowly. I'm stunned by her words. Elation is what I feel… not depression. How could they so misinterpret my disability? How could they not see how happy I am to be alive?

It was random fortune that the clot didn't break up into more pieces, didn't smash bigger parts of my brain, more functions. The surgery gave me a safe brain, a new life. I'm severely crippled, but only in this one huge way. I'm hazed by death, sideswiped. I'm quietly delirious inside not to be dead.

A clutch of close friends find my splintered speech entertaining. I hear them clucking, "Did you hear her say she has to be on her toad—her toes?"

"Did you hear that one?" They savor my ragged trials.

I call my friend "Joke," when her name is Jake. They don't let me forget how amusing my words are.

My next-door neighbor, a blustery lawyer, is outraged by their laughter.

He yells at me, "They shouldn't be making fun of you!"

"They... aren't... really," I tell him, trying to soothe his ire for me.

He doesn't get it, but I'm softened by his caring so much.

I'm like a beloved toddler who makes words, messes up, and tries again. In the messing up, family and friends applaud, laughing in pleasure. In all of my tattered, ridiculous, tragic, heroic efforts, these friends quietly see me. They take me as I am and remind me that I am still me.

My mother calls me every two or three days. The irascible, unsatisfied mother is not the one calling. This one is supportive and empathic with the ardors of getting through my day. Nearly eighty, she is sharp in mind, often too much so, cutting. She is active in social causes and gathers her energy carefully to do what she wants to do in her old New England town.

Haltingly I tell her, "I ... got up, shower...ed, had... breakfast... then......burst into tears! ... I'm exhau...sted ... it's ...only nine ... in the morning!"

She clucks sympathetically and says, "I didn't have much energy this morning either, but I wanted to clean up the leaves that have collected too long in the bottom of my yard. I raked them for a little while to do something to them. And then I sat down in a lawn chair just to look at what I did. It was good."

This picture eases me. She makes simple miseries sweet. It makes me laugh. We are two little old ladies. This sharing of infirmity feeds me, and I have a better vision of getting through each day.

I am new at this. My mother is not a graceful woman, but she models for me a certain interior grace, humor, and ease with the inconvenience of decreased ability. I can think of myself as a little old lady. A tender perspective.

Discourtesy happens all the time in New York, but some days it is unbearable. At a coffee kiosk, a window opening on the side of an old building on the Upper West Side, I open my mouth, and the few seconds I need to retrieve, "Co..ff..ee....mi...lk....., no.... sug...ar.." are too much for the vendor. "Next!" he says to the man in line on the sidewalk behind me. I'm shunted away by his curt word. The man steps easily into my place without a second thought to me and gives his order.

I'm stunned, shunned, isolated. I consider leaving. But I wait there on the street, and take the time to organize my coffee preference all over again. Ready, I step back into the front space in line and speak my order very loudly.

There is no leniency for my slowness today. I'm in tears inside. My intellect is clear, observation incisive, needs ordinary, but language is no longer there for me to express any of the assertion, anger, chutzpah.

I am an outsider in the culture of talking people around me. I understand them, but they don't hear or see me. My aphasia is a special kind of language that so few of them are willing to listen to. Inside I feel like I'm in another culture; aphasia mind is different from others. I'm an invisible stranger.

Today it is a simple cup of coffee. I stammer out the few words. But my life hammers up harshly under them.

Colleagues assure me carefully they forget words too. Their intent is to bring me into the fold of normal. But they don't lose words like I do! And I am not normal! It isn't soothing to have them discount this huge loss. There is a chasm between us. I'm standing at the other edge, and they don't want to see the breach is there. It is unnerving for them to see deeply where I am, to see the other side. No one wants to imagine not being able to talk. No one wants to the see the fragile aura of death around my halting words.

My slowness and my halting effort break up my intent. Others don't comprehend this, don't want to; it is too costly for them to be empathic. They want words to see me. I'm not seen in words. I struggle to find an essence of myself, the core without words.

A few months later, after I have naïvely restarted my small clinical practice, the irascible mother calls. She complains, "You are not doing enough for me! You are a psychologist after all!" Apparently she thinks I am well now. I steel myself to defend from her harsh words. This is familiar. I remember the cutting irritability about my shortcomings as a daughter, veiled threats of depression, the times I bit my tongue or shot out a retort. Very carefully now, I compose a defense in my mind as she rails.

Then … quite suddenly she stops … mid-sentence… Her voice gentles, "I think I don't want to continue in this direction." She begins a new sentence, on a totally different track. I am stunned by the reversal, pulling away the sharp words I have ready. My mother has simply and lightly stepped around a lifetime of entrenched hurt and walked into a new way with me. If she, if she … can do that in her seventy-ninth year of life, then it is possible for me to change anything. I can't imagine her sudden courage—in mid-sentence—to dam the torrent of years of anger and anguish. I will accept the gift, even if it is only for this moment.

But she stays with the easy comradeship and doesn't go back. The twins of death and life are entwined beneath and around our consciousness, my mother and I. We have each looked at my death, though we never speak of it. Nothing else is more important than these sweet, simple moments.

A baby research conference is being held in a big hotel in Washington, D.C., and I want to reassert this important piece of my life as it was. It is the first large research conference in the United States devoted solely to babies.

Experimental design in infant work is usually fun for me because it is so much like baby play. But now the descriptions go too fast for me to follow, and the statistical findings are too complex to grasp. In the hospital the neurologist said that I had comprehension intact, but this complexity, apparently, isn't what he meant. The clinical observation papers are easier going, sweeter, more like stories I can just ride along with.

Between sections people move into the hallways to talk together in little groups. I see colleagues I know and want to join. The verbal din of voices augments the echo in the place, and I am assailed by all of it. Quiet restaurants have gone out of vogue, and noisy ones are in, no carpets, no drapes, concrete floors, bare walls. Everyone talks louder to hear, then louder. Ordinary people have sensory screening systems to shunt the hubbub to the background and the table talk to the foreground.

The conference hallways are a loud resonant restaurant to me. I have no screening system. I talk to a colleague, the background merges into the foreground of his words. It is a jumble. My brain spins and hurts. My old shyness augments the confusion, and I haven't the endurance to push. Here in this professional place my desires for connection are lost … so lost … in the crowd of talk…. My condition shuts me out.

I look normal. No one notices the ravage inside, even those who know what has happened to me. I want to connect, go out this evening for dinner or theater. I retreat, exhausted and disappointed, to my hotel room. I fall asleep at four in the afternoon, wake at ten, call room service for a sandwich and a beer, and return to deep sleep until the next day.

After the closing morning session, I go to the National Gallery. Visually thirsty, I drink in every work of art in stunning detail, savoring it all. The patterns of color and form wash through my brain, washing out the fatigue and pain.

My eyes revel in old Indian mandalas that I paid little attention to before, tracing through the vast detail of their stories. I move eagerly along centuries of painted visions. I stay for eight hours, lunch, then dinner, barely noticing time. I have never before had this stamina in a museum.

My brain eases more and more, then becomes happy. I didn't know that a brain could be happy! Watered, refreshed, with the sweet rain of so much beauty, my brain softly laps the shores of what is.

Frustration is unvarying in my life, but I try not to focus much on it. Along with fatigue, it chokes out my flimsy path to words like brambles concealing roses. I can't afford the energy to struggle with everything, so I pull out just the brambles in front of my face. But by January, ten months after the stroke, I am flattened by fatigue.

"I must ... be depressed.... I'm... exhau...sted... all of... the time," I tell Kathy, a savvy clinician and neuropsychologist. "Maybe ... I need ... psycho....therapy!"

"You should see a speech therapist and start exercising!" She brushes off the idea of depression like dust, barely concealing her amusement.

Kathy makes pronouncements, and when she does, I do what she says. I know I'm not depressed, but I can't fathom the incessant fatigue.

By late spring I'm on my way to my first appointment with Dr. Martha Sarno, the speech pathologist Kathy selected for me. My hurrying reflection in a shop window looks like a bag lady. The clothes hang limp on her, no style. I chose them carefully this morning. Her shape is worn and bent over; her skin damp and spongy. I can almost see the grocery cart of her life's possessions. She's insubstantial, out of focus; she could blow away in a gust.

I walk into Rusk Institute for Rehabilitation, a very old hospital, feeling a bit haggard from the walk and from the window vision. I'm surrounded by yellow beige walls and hurrying people. I'm disoriented. I struggle to stay composed. I approach a uniformed guard and I'm slow to speak. He asks who I want to see and I stammer her name. He smiles cheerily, points to the elevators down the noisy hall, and tells me the floor number. I go up the elevator as he said and ask the only person in an empty and suddenly quiet hallway. She points, no words, down the hall, gestures left around a corner.

I find a tiny office and a secretary. I wait standing, and then Dr. Sarno appears to greet me, a formal but welcoming smile. I like her already, in her tailored feminine ivory colored suit with a flared skirt. She is the Director of

Speech and Language Pathology. Much later I learn she began the department at Rusk, created modern speech rehabilitation, and was awarded a honorary doctor of medicine from the University of Goteborg, Sweden.

At first her office looks small and nondescript, but entering, I see it is wrapped around the edge of the building, with huge windows looking high over the city. I'm in a spacious tower.

She is listening carefully as I rush haltingly to tell my medical story, then how tired I am all the time with my practice. At length, I am spent.

Gently she tells me, "You are imploding yourself with language in trying to do a clinical practice. You're exhausted because you are trying to do what you can't do!"

My body, straining to attend to her words, relaxes its grip. "S..o...! That's all ... it is!" I think. Suddenly I feel euphoric; it seems possible now.

"Most aphasics with the kind of insult you had don't continue in high verbal professions like yours." There isn't anything dreadfully wrong, only that I am trying to go beyond what my damaged brain can manage. She does not dissuade me from continuing my practice. "I'm thinking how it would be for me as an academic," she continues. She speaks as though she has been in my place. She penetrates my desires and my losses and takes me far beyond the reflection of the worn bag lady. I feel seen, with all the pieces of me disarrayed before her.

"One recovers from stroke. One doesn't recover from aphasia, but, rather, with aphasia," she says.

I won't be "cured," I think. This is curiously reassuring and feels like she has spoken my reality. Live with it, not against or despite it, as I have been doing.

"Do any of the arts that please you, and do them a lot," she tells me. I didn't expect this; she has handed me an immense gift. I imagine her words written on a prescription pad.

She shows me how to set practical priorities carefully and often simply do less. I space my few office sessions over the day, allowing time in between to do non-verbal activities, listen to music, look at art, do hand work, exercise, or simply rest. The mindfulness of choosing and streamlining does allow me ease to see patients and have more pleasure. Less is more.

As with the neurosurgeon, I feel I am in the presence of great simplicity, depth of seeing. Her words open doorways of possibility for me. She is practical and magical at once.

She has shown me signs for this road, the expanses as well as the potholes. She mentors me over months and then years. I get a little better. I do more, then have new bouts of crushing fatigue. I am happy in what I am doing, and two days later the fatigue socks in like a dense fog. I am surprised every time, not seeing it coming. This mindfulness is a deeper practice than I think.

PART TWO:
WALK IN WILDERNESS

I dare to register at Parson's School of Design. I have no pretensions to art, no talent, as it were. Go to the best to start on the prescription Dr. Sarno gave me, I think. I'm anxious speaking to strangers by myself, and I feel like an art dunce with real art students.

Knowing so little, I choose Color Theory, then fear it will be wordy. We sit at tables arranged in a large circle with fat bundles of 4x6 inch silk-screen color swatches, scissors, and glue. The colors are textured and luscious to the eye. We spend our time cutting up the colors, working out little exercises. We learn the brashness of comple-mentary colors, how any color looks different beside any other, how you think you are going to get one effect and you get another. I find pleasure in the simplicity and challenge of the visual.

The instructor walks around the inside of the circle of tables commenting and critiquing. He nods appreciatively one day at my work as he goes around the oval, "That's the work of a mature person. You know what you are about." I'm startled.

Next I choose a flower drawing class. In all those summers of drawing, I could never translate what I did to my life in the city. Whatever creativity I had stayed with the weeds and wild flowers on that small island.

A vase of flowers sits in the center of the table we sit around, each week a different bouquet, sometimes exotic, sometimes common. The bouquet as a whole is too

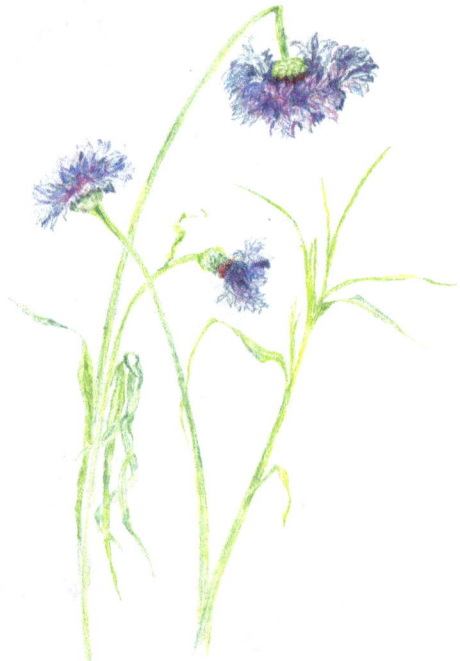

complex to me, so I choose two or three blossoms and immerse my eyes in the individual qualities of each. The bent stem of one leans over, casually drifts in space. The fluffy edge of a purple aster is disfigured with yellow, secreting its mortality inside its beauty.

I pare the overabundance of leaves to a few that urge brightly or quiver around themselves, no vase. My flowers are suspended across the page.

I take a break and walk around the room to look at everyone else's work. I see enormous differences. One woman draws her blossoms in a long row growing out of the bottom of the paper. I find it very odd and childish. But the judgment recedes, and I see the pleasure in her radical arrangement; her use of the colored pencils is sharp and bold. I am more tentative. I learn from her.

The teacher hangs our work on the wall for the last twenty minutes of each class. She doesn't critique so much as appreciate. She describes the special way each of us looked at the same vase of flowers and then set a unique vision onto the paper. She is supportive of what we see.

This is a profound lesson for me, this intimate act of private seeing. No "right" way, only the personal way.

My seeing is changing. A new kind of candor emerging.

Everywhere I listen to music—in the streets, on the subway, and especially between patients. I plug a baroque chamber sound-scape into my headphones, and the outside chaotic sounds and energies of the city disengage from my body. My brain floats free in Hayden or Corelli. The sound is intimate, resonant against the battered walls of my aching brain. It smoothes on like a salve, and my verbal brain quiets in the surround—as if the Dalai Lama is chanting.

I have believed that words, good sturdy words, were core to my existence. To articulate thought well is to be alive, to be seen in the world. I am learning other ways of being. From drawing I ease into watercolor painting, tiny brushes and delicate forms, a cluster of daisies with pinks and burnished purples.

A classmate urges me to try a class at the Art Students League, a room filled with flowers. I'm arrested by this vision. The reality, even more than I thought, overflows with abundance, flowers everywhere. An assistant hands me a book illustrating different botanical kinds of leaves, tells me to practice them over and over and be accurate. Being more casual, I have trouble copying. Another day I learn how to wet the paper so that the color blows out when it is very wet and becomes more defined as the paper dries. I'm eager to experiment.

I begin a lavender chrysanthemum from the flowers around me. I can't imagine doing this bountiful flower all in one color; so I use different colors, blues and some reds, to create contrast and shadow. I'm pleased with my cunning. One of the two teachers comes by and I expect a little bit of praise; instead she says, "You can't do it that way!" and walks abruptly onto the next student. I am startled in my bones.

I may lose the delicate seeing that has been emerging if I stay here. I could be smothered in technique. Something about my life is at stake. I have to trust something new in myself… I revel in the sensual beauty of the flowered room, but I must leave. I mustn't cage my own way of expressing, however unsure and untutored it is.

Aphasia is a group of language disorders that often follow a stroke, or brain trauma like an accident, or diseases affecting the brain. The main aphasias are expressive and receptive aphasia. I have expressive aphasia, difficulty retrieving words. I am slow and halting. In receptive aphasia people have difficulty understanding words they hear, slow in putting them together. There is a third, primary progressive aphasia, a rare form of expressive aphasia that comes on slowly without a precipitating incident.

My mind beyond language is otherwise intact, an irritating but common paradox. Words are so lacking—sometimes dimwitted—but the thinking, observing mind is sharp and clear. For me, I am living my childhood fear that I would be found out as dumb. Here it is. I must climb around it.

One of Dr. Sarno's people gives me many little standard language tests. "Say words beginning with B, and I will time you."

"Boy, bone," I say and I get stuck on using the same vowel o. I can't think of any more words with it, and I don't think of using another vowel, like e or a. I know this should be easy, and I sweat as the seconds of my silence roll by. I am asked for names of animals, and the same thing happens, two or three and I am stuck in silence.

The tests confirm my functioning as "high level" expressive aphasia, as the doctors told me in the hospital. I am impaired in retrieving words and in fluency. I have no impairment in comprehension on the simple tasks of the tests, unlike most people with aphasia who have a combination. Nevertheless I am not good at understanding complex language, like the research talks. Comparing my scores with adults who haven't had a stroke, my fluency is "very low" normal, rather like the language of a slow child.

Being told early on that I was a "high level" aphasic and wouldn't need therapy unfortunately gave me the impression that my impairments were smaller than they actually were. I thought I could navigate the recovery landscape alone. Instead I had to bump and careen around rutted, potholed roads to learn otherwise. I needed a lot more information to learn this new landscape.

Two years after the stroke I am still locked in pursuit of writing the paper I started on the summertime island, a test of my conceptual mind. It is a practical matter; how much of my professional self is gone?

This touches deeply into my psyche. I was a shy child after my parents separated, when I was four. My mother was depressed for years, and my father was lost to me. My older brother, the smart one, was the star. I loved him and felt unseen by my parents, undernourished. Going to kindergarten when I was still four was another loss I didn't begin to make up until I was in the sixth grade, when Mrs. Mortenson read poetry and showed us paintings—The Dance of the Nymphs. I came alive, and I loved her. Still it was a long path to discover I had a mind.

Stan Grand continues his interest, works patiently with me on the paper. It is a constant strain to fit word to idea, then rearrange everything to shape idea to vision with him, returning over and over to fit word to word. I am in a fevered passion to return to verbal culture, to return to a professional culture of abstraction and be admitted as an equal.

Through high school and college I struggled with finding words, hoped I had something to say. I took debate and dramatics to push myself into expression. Language seemed to obscure what was inside, not illuminate. Losing speech when I thought I had stepped so far out of all of that, brought it all back. I recognize myself in the loss of speech; it is not altogether new. It isn't the same now, but somehow familiar enough.

Between us, Stan and I have made a wonderful paper. I see that my mind works even though my words are scrappy and not fluent. In fact, I am ecstatic beyond reason, extravagantly expansive with relief. A part of my fractured self has been sewn back together through the careful stitching and tailoring of this paper.

Another close colleague, Norbert Freedman, urges us to present the paper at one of the psychoanalytic institutes, IPTAR. I can't understand what I read when I read out loud, and I can't read with expression. But there is no question in my mind. I will read the paper!

I fashion a kind of musical notation on the manuscript, marking cues for slowing, speeding up, emphasis, pausing, even the rising and falling of my voice, throughout the manuscript.

"Historically psychoanalysis has insisted on the maintenance of an integrative view among the biological, the psychosocial, and the social contributors to the development of object relations. In this paper, we shall present the beginning phase of a remarkable treatment of an autistic baby…"

I practice the script again and again … and yet again … carefully following the notations of expression to make sure the reading is well done. I can hear when the expression I want is right. Something musical. But I know when I read to an audience I will have no idea what it means. I am compelled. It has it to be impeccable and engaging.

The institute arranges a small lecture hall for an intimate turnout. The room fills, and fills more. People stand in the doorways, the aisles, then out into the halls. It will be many years later before I understand that they have come for me!

At the last nervous moment, I arrange a fail-safe with Stan to hand it over smoothly to him if I can't finish it by myself. I do read to the end with all the élan and beauty that I intended! I have carefully cobbled together a voice and knocked on the door of my professional community. For a moment there at the podium, I can see my full self through the wreckage. Colleagues cluster about me with praise. I am seen.

Later the paper is published. I write more papers, always with colleagues. The effort for me is huge. I am desperate to be seen, not trusting the first success.

My Parsons flower drawing teacher, after many semesters with her, is leaving teaching. Like me, she is balancing her life and work with a disability, multiple sclerosis. She is leaving to concentrate on her textile design work. When I ask for a reference, she sends me to her own painting teacher.

Henry Pearson, a well-known painter, neither shows his work or anyone else's when he teaches. He quietly persists in our finding our own style. In the first class he talks practicals about materials, and that's the end of class teaching.

Instead he sits down with every one of us individually during the class, talks about poetry, movies, what I am doing or what I want to do, in my life or in my painting. If I want him to give me technical instruction, he will give only what I ask for. He creates an atmosphere of ease and expression, wandering in personal experiment—seeing in the mind. Some students are painting in oils and others in watercolor. Some are doing collage, and still others are sculpting, though the class is titled "Abstract Watercolor."

I don't know what I want to do, let alone how to experiment. Most of the new people drop out by the third week. The rest are old-timers, some of many years. I stay, not knowing why.

Without class assignments, I bring my vase of flowers. I am comfortable here, the students companionable. The three women at my table work in totally different styles, and it's a lesson just watching how they work. One is a mathematics teacher and works with webs of grids. Another paints in geometric spirals on a small canvas, changing the colors in small spaces each time she goes around. Though I am intimidated, it is the right place to be.

Henry has an ability to see beyond what I am doing. He offers visions to tweak my imagination. One day in my second year with him, he lends me a book of Japanese paintings.

"Here, Ruth, look at these. Find the work that is like yours."

I take the book home, delight in the misty, the spare, the ornate. The skill is awesome. Whatever can he be thinking? Over and over I look. I don't find anything remotely like my work.

Sheepish, I say to him, "I can't find what you mean."

He shows me a corner of a painting, simple, messy rocks lying in a stream.

I am so touched, I stop my flirtation with fragile and delicate, the incandescent light of a fragile peach, the delicacy of a bunch of leeks, or the pattern of pink and yellow tulips blended across the page.

I begin to embrace bold and move toward messy. Working with less order and more abandon is hard to do, and it takes me a long time. Meanwhile the pieces of paper I work on get bigger and bigger. The flowers get larger, more voluptuous, and less tied to the specifics of the flower. Now they are flowers in my mind without a vase.

It is here I begin to follow the thread of my own seeing. It isn't a conscious intellectual seeing. It emerges out of my body. Henry is a canny mentor in this. He sits by me and shows me what my mind's eye is looking at, presses me beyond.

The painting has become more than speech therapy.

One afternoon I'm so exhausted I can't drag my body out the door to class. But I must paint! In my small galley kitchen looking out over silvered rooftops below, I jerry-rig a place to work. The half-elephant size paper is beautiful, heavy and coarse to the touch. The first gesture, a setting for everything else, is clumsy and artless. I scrub it out and create more mess.

The paper is expensive, but I begin again with a new piece. I have a vision of swirling patterns, poinsettia leaves with their tiny, orangey flowerets in the center. I paint the veins of the leaves in wide gestures of blue-reds, orangey-reds, purples, splotches of white paper showing through. With a carbon pencil I harshly trace the swirls of leaves now flowing around the coarse paper. It is the vision I had, but wilder and rougher in the actuality. The next day I put in a dense vegetative background of browns, greens, and black to complete the painting. The background is a new experiment, and it works.

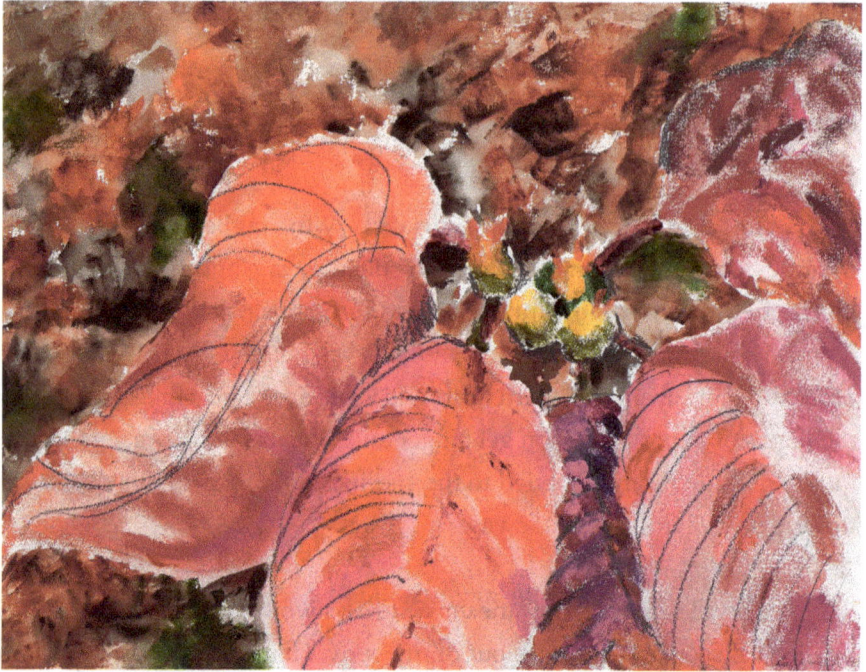

I paint from the terrible damage to my brain. The intensity of fatigue flows through arms and hands, becomes passion on the paper. I paint strongly into rest, into the joy of being alive, into the urgency to speak, to see patients anyway.

Death slammed my brain, marking its presence there, and thrust me into life.

I have crossed a border. I have become a painter.

Over time I become boldly gestural, no brushes, just rags. I discover black as an actual color, not negative, not a depressive allusion. Black is vibrant and fertile; my death lives there, holding the whole composition together, and the risky, vibrant, passionate reds circle its center. Red tulips travel up the paper in angled lines surrounded by soft yellow and white blossoms, the paper wetted to soften edges, at once creating bold and ethereal.

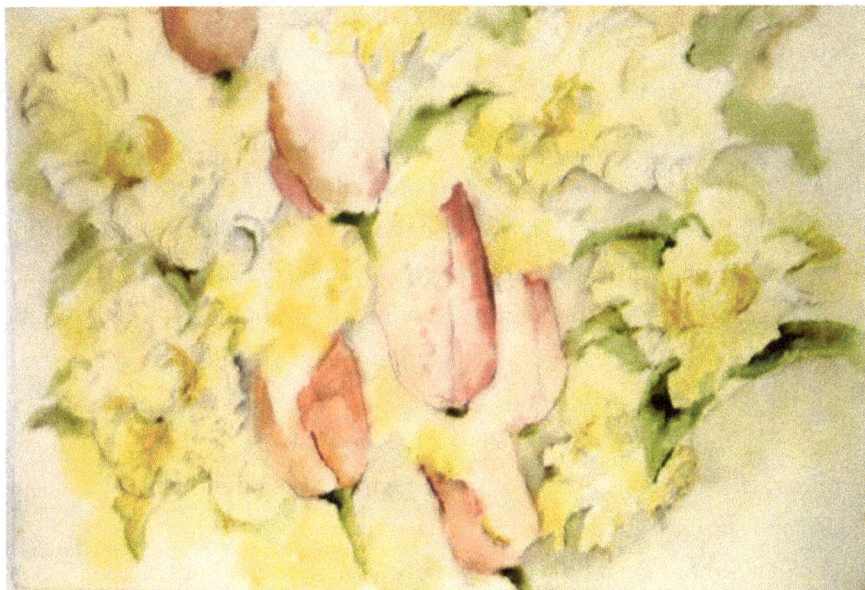

I come to class left-brain exhausted, and when I leave after three hours, I am rested and exhilarated. Although my speech is halting, my brain feels balanced when I leave… and I am happy. At the heart of this balance is the creation of pleasure, which is the center of this life of recovery. If I love something, I do it. If there is pleasure, then I can persevere into what is difficult.

I'm challenging and enlivening my right brain to express beauty in what I can do. My beleaguered verbal left brain turns down its rush to words and finds profound rest. The impairments soften.

I take paint and drawing material wherever I go. After a conference in Europe reading the paper, I go to the Tate Museum in London.

I have overdone my left-brain at the conference. So I look at all the paintings in the many galleries, again as though quenching thirst, falling into pools of detail. My eyes fill with images of draping: the fall of a cloth from a round table, the draping of a woman's skirt and shawl in a Victorian drawing room, the folds of a man's breeches. I find pleasure even in the huge voluptuous Renaissance paintings that I usually pass by.

I go out into one of those little London parks where groups of people lounge in the summertime grass. Inspired by what I have seen in the Tate, I look at how clothes fall on people's bodies as they sit in the mild sunshine, at how the clothes are billowy, how the shadows fall on the fabrics. I make little sketches, playing with the details, how the draping defines a body. These are experiments; I haven't done figure drawing before, but I'm thirsty from the luscious details my eyes and mind found in the museum.

At home I do quick sketches of people on the subway. Shoes are wonderfully intimate and unobtrusive to draw. The ones that attract me are worn and scrubby and tell stories of hard living.

Sometimes I am a little bolder. I draw the draping lines of a ski jacket. I try to remember later the arc of a woman's back, a textured, heavy coat shaping itself over her stooping body in an intimate oval. I look at what happens to the flowers in a black printed dress as a woman folds her body down on a park bench.

The seeing is what delights me; I am beginning to partner with my brain.

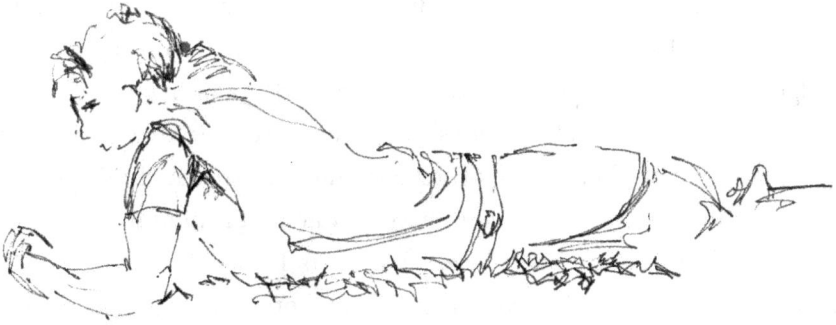

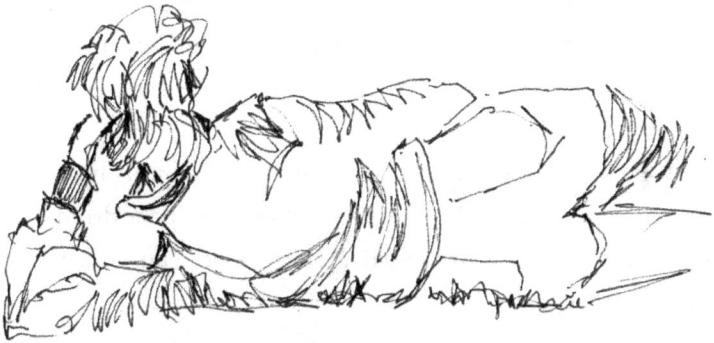

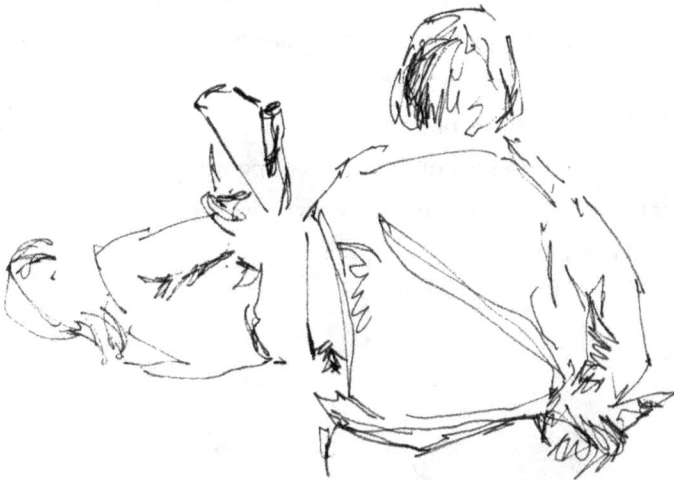

My relationship with George planted the seeds of seeing. On our first date he took me walking on Brooklyn Bridge, the wooden walkway suspended high between the lanes of traffic. He drew my attention to the magic of the bridge, the art of it. His visions of pattern, form, and motion in the walking led my eyes into his. I fell in love with seeing, with the bridge, and with him.

He made fine photographs of architectural details of the city, developing and carefully printing them in a tiny, cold-water flat behind the wholesale meat markets on Gansevoort Street. For years I stood beside him in the darkroom, in whatever place we lived, while he worked the enlarger, intuiting the right amount of light, dodging in areas, holding others. I listened to him count the seconds in the developer and heave it out, confident in the right densities of blacks and grays. When the image came up in the last solution, I heard his verdict, wondered at his precision, wondered how he came to his vision for this piece.

Being in the darkroom with him was like sitting by the drum, listening, watching, waiting for the time to become one with the drum. I saw greatness in his vision. He loved what he saw. I learned the beauty and the resourcefulness of the process he wove.

A few years after the stroke, my daughter invites me to go with her to a Robert Bly conference with poets and Jungians and a lot of complex talk. So much listening undoes my verbal brain, and I escape to the surrounding woods. I make little paintings of granite rocks, loamy forest floor, nestled weeds. Without being conscious of the Japanese painting of rocks in a steam that Henry Pearson showed me, I make my own vision of careless, handsome rocks among the trees.

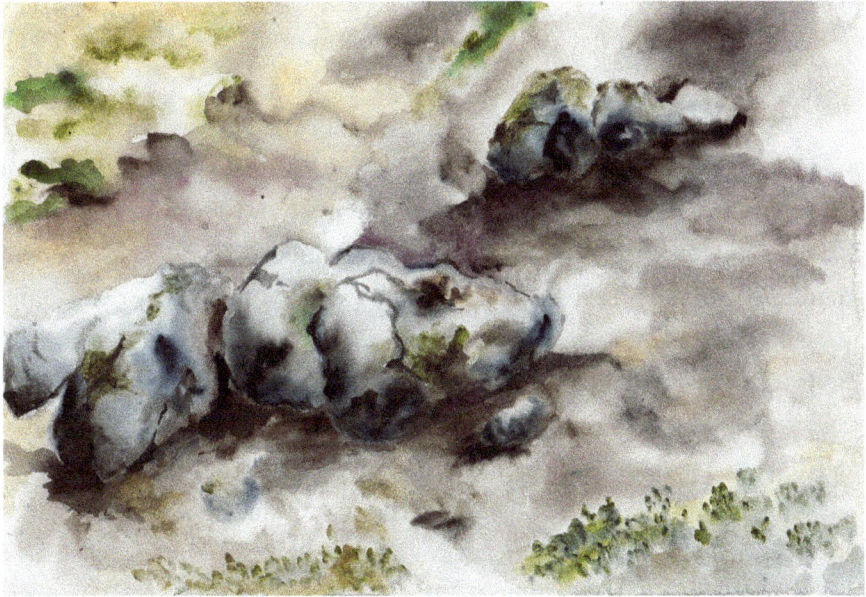

My mind calms as my seeing and my spirit extend out into the woods. I am seeing life … in fewer words. I feel what I see. I am in a nether world between speech and no speech. I am not conscious of the power of what is happening, how I am being shaped new.

In the fourth year after the stroke, I mumble to friends about finding a job.

They try not to laugh, but I need more collegiality. One of them invites me to volunteer at the cancer hospital where she is on the faculty. This I can do. I think that I am a natural to do psychotherapy with cancer patients. It is a teaching hospital and none of the adult psychotherapy services want a volunteer encroach¬ing on their turf. In an interview with the chief psychiatrist in pediatrics, Dr. Yehuda Nir, I mention my baby specialty in passing. He lights up. "We don't have one of you!" he says, delighted. No one else wants the turf of children who don't yet talk—babies and toddlers under two. In fact I am horrified that babies are dying of cancer. But I'm in my element with my box of baby evaluation toys, my non-verbal communication with babies.

Oddly I am not depressed by this work, rather I'm comfortable being in that chancy mortal place with these mothers. In fact, I feel inordinate joy. It is my nearness to my own death that connects me deeply to the hearts of these women who are living, fearfully and hopefully, at the edge of life and death every day with their babies. Yehuda Nir gives me constant enthusiastic support for these unusual talents and mentors me in how to hold in myself the reality of the fragility of life and death here.

I speak to the mothers about how they hold their babies in love and life, at the same time releasing them in love to the possibility of death. I give voice and acknowledge the tightrope they live on. The brisk progression of ordinary infant development is a resource in illness to support health. I show the mothers how to use the baby's natural development through gentle but challenging play.

A mother and toddler are both afraid because of the fragility of the little girl's health, so she doesn't walk. She can be sick and walk too, I tell the mother. With soft patience I soothe both of them into the mysterious delight of walking.

I hold the baby's body securely as a foot floats near the floor. It waivers in fear, barely touching. Subtly I drop her weight into her feet and she feels the floor firmly. She is surprised. Standing with both feet, still held strongly in my arms, she takes the first challenging and magical step onto the floor. Neither mother nor staff can believe it's happening. Mother walks the IV pole beside us, and I support the toddler's walk down the hallway. They practice in the following days, both delighting in this milestone. A kind of robust health is taking place between them that helps sturdy them in facing the illness issues more securely. Early development is a powerful force, a driver for change, and I use it here.

Infants, at the get-go, love novelty. The developing brain recognizes the familiar and then chooses the new. A related interest is variety. They are the way the brain develops. Variety is also how my brain is developing, seeing art in museums, looking at the world visually — people's costuming, the way vegetables are laid out, the light flowing across the violets in my lawn this morning.

Variety is also sensing something more about the non-verbal here with these babies, the sense of a baby's vitality, how much communication there is in them, the visual, sensory quality of it.

Variety and pleasure in whatever I am doing makes my rush to return to the verbal world much more tolerable. They make my stay here in the in-between world richly engrossing. At Parsons I feel the visual sensations of the paint moving across the paper, and the feeling comes with me as I watch each baby and mother struggle across a canvas of life and death. The layers of grief in my own body find affinities with a mother's anguish in holding life for her baby. I can't clearly articulate any of this yet, but I'm beginning to sense how my body's limitations help me see.

I scrub and gown-up to be sterile to go into a reverse isolation unit to be with a baby boy who was born with no immune system. To keep him alive he is being protected from the world's germs and viruses in this sterile little room. Today he has just had a painful bath. He is crying from the irritation of the water and the cloth washing his rashy delicate skin. The nurse dries him off and wraps a warm blanket around him.

She gladly hands him off to me, assuring me he will continue his fretful crying. She leaves. I sit in the room's rocking chair and cuddle him into my body, gently rock him, and begin softly singing. My body remembers how good this feels, a baby tucked warm in my arms. He snuggles into me, softening his chuffing and crying. He quiets as I rock and continue my little songs. I can't sing since my surgery, but I can sing quietly to him. The sudden quiet alarms the nurse outside who comes to the door: "Is he dead?"

Only the ordinary sleep of a peaceful baby.

Yehuda tells me it is time for me to attend in the death of one of my baby patients. "An essential initiation," he says. "You must do this!" A baby's death is too much to bear, and I am apprehensive.

I'm seeing a toddler and his grandmother, showing them both gentle ways to play. It doesn't help much as he gets sicker and weaker, less able to hold attention to the outside or to toys. His grandmother bonds strongly with me, talks about her passionate desire to see him well. I see his little body bundled up in a little wagon, rag doll arms hanging out as she pulls him around the halls and sometimes lets him sit there outside his room. She so much wants life for him, even the little shreds here in the hall. I too want him to live, but his life is ebbing away, not to be so for either grandmother or me. He is holding this thread of life for her. It is her love and her insistence on life that he holds onto. This is clear to the nurses now. And I see that.

He's very weak. It is time for him to be able to go out of this life. Nurses, a social worker, and I are here in his room with her to support her gently, to help him. She is not ready. She holds him tightly to her breast. One and then another of us take him to hold. I sit beside her, telling her quietly how heroic she has been to mother this baby when her own daughter couldn't. She alone has given him the gift of mothering.

Gradually, very gradually, I speak of how letting him go is the biggest and hardest act of love, not a failure of love. He needs her love in order go; he needs her to say it is OK. Someone hands the baby back to her. She takes a long moment, looks at him carefully, and tells him how very much she loves him—and that it is all right for him to go. She holds herself steady in her love for him. He sighs, his body relaxes. We continue to sit quietly with her. The room changes around us—the baby energy that had suffused it is gone.

My mother, resting on her couch in midday, dies swiftly, unexpectedly, of a heart attack. Milk is heating on the stove for her favorite cocoa. The man who does her lawn has looked in on her. When the Lexington police call me, I run screaming around my apartment. I can't bear the loss of the lovely companionship we've had. She's left my life too soon.

She has a big white angora cat she calls Kitty, who escapes from her house in a mad rush when anyone comes to visit. She and Kitty have an affection based on shared aloofness. When I settle into my mother's house that evening, Kitty crouches slowly from the kitchen like she is stalking prey. She turns her white head from side to side. Her big, wide black eyes look carefully all around the room. Then she focuses intensely on me, as if to say, "She's gone, isn't she!?"

"Yes," I say, "she is gone, and I am here. I belonged to her too."

Kitty, who has never stayed in the same room with me, now settles herself on the couch across from me. I'm relieved to have company in this house of death. We sit the long night together sharing our loss.

Carrying the box of my mother's ashes a few days later, I meet my daughter, my brother and his wife, and my mother's friends at the cemetery gate, and together we walk along the rambling paths through the trees to a place I found under a sprawling old tree. She wanted her body to nourish trees, and so it will. Her minister is gone for the summer, so I decide to I lead the simple ritual burial myself, rather than leave it all to the student minister.

Most of my life my relationship to my mother was ambivalent, frequently harshly so. Her irritability and inner discontent often made loving her and feeling loved by her unmanageable. I had sometimes imagined I would be relieved when she died.

The time of willing companionship she made with me in the short time since my stroke is an offering to my life beyond any words I can say today. Yet I do reflect on her surprising lifelong capacity to struggle with herself and to live a significant life. In the certainty of grief, I am poignantly proud of her.

My self is in transition. It is a long time before I understand that I lost more than expressive words, but a syntax that goes with them: the structures that put things together that are narrative cohesion. I lost the planning parts of language, which are essential to intention and action. My relationship to time and space was subtly changed. But I don't know about this now.

The connectors of mind to life's activity are the sounds of the world and the communicative sounds with self and community, whether human or animal. Effective functioning in the world is related to the syntax of the communicative sounds, inner and outer.

When I lost so much of my expressive verbal mind, I lost part of the subtle behavioral syntax attached to it. In struggling to re-grow the expressive, I had also to re-grow the syntactic connections to daily functioning. An example: I used to have a big pouch over my shoulder as a pocketbook in which it was easy to fumble around with my hands, sight unseen, and find whatever I wanted. Now I can't do that; such a small task with its hidden uncertainty drives me anxious. I am lost.

A consultant tells me to buy a bag with many pockets and with many little bags inside. Then I organize the "stuff" so that I know where everything is, and return it there after using. This seems simpleminded, and it is for an ordinary brain, and may seem of little consequence. But in losing language, I also lost how language connects me to intention and planning in my life, unhinging ordinary parts of my daily life.

I have to be more deliberate now about where I am going, in space, specifying sequences in directions for myself to get there. I am easily confused by the complexity of my environment, sights and sounds, less able to keep focus now. I don't really notice this day to day and can't articulate it until much later, but the loss of these connections is an undercurrent that make my life as difficult as it is. The great exhaustion I experience is not just, then, production of words and sentences. It is also the functional limitations I have now of trying to plan and run a normally complex life.

So there are syntactic relationships in verbal mind and perhaps analogous codes in body functioning. Like most modern Western people, I don't live much in my body and live very much in my head. So I haven't much resource available from the sensory codes in my body to support and do fill-in for this new loss. I can barely articulate what is happening there, and that is the crux of it.

Art and music not only become places of rest and balance, they are also significant routes for me to develop non-linear sensory sequencing in my daily activity.

As human beings, especially in Western culture, we are run by verbal language, too much believing the layers of its meanings, perhaps acting too much by its allusions. With not enough words, I am both pulled back into language to fit into community and simultaneously drawn out of it to see and think beyond language where there is more ease for me.

The sensory life of babies, their vitalities of articulate communication before language, the cogent visual and aural experiences of art and music unrestricted by language structures or associations, the fundamental reality of death in my body that survived to know what being alive is: all these have become the beginnings, models of different ways of being in the world for me.

I am moving further and further in the direction of living in sensory and non-verbal worlds. The wealth of sensation, reception, and communication in the unconscious meets the conscious brain's aptitudes to walk in other worlds, to know altered states of mind, and to be in service in different ways, without so many words.

After a few years my little world of closest friends feels too small, and I want to expand my circle. A new friend invites me to her Upper West Side dinner party. There are two couples, my friend's husband, and me in the living room. We've been comfortably settled on cushy couches and served drinks. My friend is in the kitchen preparing dinner. I know none of the people around me. Introductions have been cursory. There has been no personal getting acquainted chat; everyone else seems to know one another.

The conversation moves too rapidly for me. Someone is talking about business, and someone else picks up a tangential thought and veers off to the economy, and from there it goes to fashion. I am listening very carefully, trying to put a few words together to respond into the flow of the smart conviviality. By the time I do put together the few words to speak, several topics have already gone by, and I am too late. I can't just jump back three topics and enter; I don't have a segue of words to do that. It is a blur. No one notices. No one takes an interest in the quiet woman off to the side.

Everything changes in the dining room. My friend is careful to circulate the conversation around the sparkling, beautifully laid table so no one is left out. The talk is bright, intellectual, thoughtful, funny. I am enjoying myself. Everyone is having a turn. Recent news in the papers about scandal in foster care comes up, so my friend turns to me identifying me as the child specialist.

Instantly I'm in the crosshairs. I must say something reasonably intelligent, but the politics and the human needs of the distressed system are overwhelmingly complex. I could manage a thought about some elegant piece of it. Then I realize with horror that I will have to sustain some compelling discussion. I can't actually do any of those things. Even this far out from the stroke, I can't open the black box of words at will. I lose verbal presence when I'm in the limelight. I'm in a quandary.

The moment lengthens, and my stress soars. I decide to say something banal to get off the verbal hook. I say mildly, "What a muddle!" The faces around me are blank. The silence is so deep it is scary. I am falling ... falling through the cracks. I wish desperately to say, "Yes, yes, I am one of you. I am intelligent inside here. I want you to know that!" But I haven't the words. No one knows my inner peril but my friend, who does doesn't help me out.

I had, in fact, worked in the foster care system years ago and could have much to say. Like the foster care system, my being here in this dining room is overwhelming. I can't find my way around in it.

A woman down the table smoothes over the awkward moment by shifting the topic to a book she is reading. I've made an unpleasantness in the evening, and I'm cast aside, not spoken to again. The heavy brown door of the apartment closes behind me when I leave, distraught.

I'm taking a last walk the whole length of the Promenade along the edge of Brooklyn Heights. It's the top shelf of the stacked lanes of the Brooklyn-Queens Expressway. The clamor of the traffic below is hidden from the quiet neighborhood above. Walking the cobblestones with Jake today, I feel as layered as the city. I drink in the gardens and back facades of the elegant nineteenth-century townhouses, stealing a glimpse of the panoramic view from their windows as we stroll.

My health is a shambles, lungs in constant painful flames. First it was the winter bronchitis, and then the summertime. I knew after the stroke my days were numbered in this chaotic, noisy, ultra-verbal city.

I am too sick to continue here now. No matter what I want, I have to leave. I've found a group clinical practice in the Pacific Northwest a couple of hours from where my daughter lives, and I'm leaving to join them.

As we walk the Promenade I think of the Fourth of July. Thousands of people come from all across Brooklyn to see fireworks at the Statue of Liberty across the Bay. They pack themselves gently. The "ooos" and "aaahhs" flow as one voice through the crowd. At the end there is a sweet urban festive air, no mugging, no conflict. It is a democratic place, this Promenade.

As a young woman I loved the roar and buzz, mystery and elegance of New York, but it was also a difficult city for a girl from Omaha. The dirt, the smell after a garbage strike, the disheveled buildings, the poverty, and the careless anonymity were bruising. For all its paradox, it is where I have lived for the last thirty years. I married, worked, had a baby, divorced, succeeded with graduate school, made a career. The city is my home. And now I am leaving.

The immensity of Lower Manhattan spreads before me as I look toward Brooklyn Bridge knitting its cables across to City Hall Park. I am stepping off the cliffs of this city and my life here. It is not courage. It's like the surgery, no choice. Choose life. Choose to protect my body.

I am flowing west in a perplexing mix of joy and sorrow. The journey feels shrouded as I step onto the airplane; I don't know what I will find.

I'm in a culture shock I don't expect. My body is conditioned to hunker down to urban sensations: tight spaces, canyons of buildings, and stimulating streets. Here in the Pacific Northwest my body is assailed by the expansiveness of the space: broad valleys, chains of mountains, wide skies, and quieter towns. My body feels small, unbalanced in this scale.

Rhododendrons grow lush and rampant, unlike the delicate laurel, its relative in the East. Fir trees soar higher than I've ever seen. The mystical and the magical seem alive in this landscape: rocks, trees, birds flying across the sky. Its palpable magic whispers to me of the older indigenous culture suffusing the air and earth.

The place feels like Greece, where my daughter and I traveled to celebrate her graduation from college. There the land and the sky seemed stark and portentous, mythic in scope. We walked in the cave of the god Zeus, saw ruins of temples in ordinary backyards. I stood on a stone rampart one afternoon and felt like Odysseus reading portents in the hawk silhouette that rode high into the pallid sky. I noticed a bird skating off a ledge below me, and it felt fraught with meaning.

Now here in the Pacific Northwest the land speaks in softer tones, more nuanced voices than Greece. But as there, I listen and watch.

I've found an apartment in a little harbor town on Puget Sound. I can see a brilliant slice of the glacial top of Mt. Rainier from its balcony. Down the hill three blocks, I sit after work with my feet up on a wooden porch railing behind a restaurant and watch the harbor traffic. Sailboats, working boats, rowboats ply from one side to the other, in and out of the harbor, reminding me of summer vacations in Maine. There as here, I glimpse the social mores of small town life. It is high summer, late afternoon, and the slanting, glistening light brings everything into sharp relief. I am not on vacation.

I turn a bedroom into my first art studio here in this apartment—unheard of luxury to urban me. With a studio I become independent in my art, working without a class, drawing and painting at my whim, my desire.

Leigh, the office manager of the practice I've joined, went to Antioch College like me but more than a decade later. She is tall, lanky, and full of zest, and when we meet says, "I've been so eager to see you, woman from New York, woman from Antioch!" She is infectious. I feel instant affinity. We are both artists. She is rowdy and compulsive in her art; she tweaks me beyond my ways of seeing.

Her husband is dying of cancer, another deeper bond. I meet him once for tea at their home on a little island in the Sound. We stroll through their gardens, admire vegetables, sunflowers, and tall clusters of poppies. The day is softly sunny, so we walk along the water's edge through new young trees. He is weak and becomes chilled. Leigh goes back to the house for a jacket. When she is out of earshot, he presses me quietly. "Ruth, I want you to make sure she follows her art. It is her path. I've kept her from it."

With breathtaking courage, she tends him all the way through his dying. And then she is off and running with art, with me on her tail. We take life drawing and clay sculpture classes in the small community college art department, a little hidden jewel. We are a bold duo among the tentative young students, and the contrast makes me even more audacious. Leigh's rowdy side is a good influence on me. I plunge into new media: ceramic sculpture, monoprints, pushing past the technical to find my own voice.

On a trip to New York I spend an afternoon with Henry in his tiny apartment/studio, bringing new work to show him. At length he says of a color pencil portrait of Leigh, "You are a good observer, Ruth. Now bring something unique into what you see." I thought I had; he pushes me deeper.

At home I drop into easy experimentation, a playful, unconstrained self without words. With this new freedom I lose self-consciousness in my art, the bedrock of my brain's balance, its rest and peace. Challenge and play make my brain more flexible—and yes, happy.

I am often homesick for New York friends, museums, galleries, and music—yes, and the tumult, the dirt, and the sophistication. Invisibility and isolation remain issues in my life here, but less so. My body and brain don't have to work quite so hard to maintain.

In a clay sculpture class I form a figure of a woman, none of the fine molding of bone and muscle the professor is teaching us. I make her rough and primitive with wings coming from her shoulders; she is running, a banner flying across her breast. She becomes a gift for my daughter to celebrate her graduate degree.

Remembering the book of Japanese paintings of many paneled works that Henry showed me back in his class, I take up the challenge of painting trios or quartets. Each of the panels must stand alone as a composition while the group unifies into a larger image. On the floor in my studio, I'm on my knees to make a quartet. Three panels of four come easily, the last one is difficult. I have to redo it over and over, faltering over pulling together the abstract flower forms. Finally the fourth one settles in as though it were thought from the beginning; the four are successfully one.

Flower forms surge and spiral in the paintings I make now. They are increasingly abstract, loosening, becoming more gestural. I play at constructing little foam sculptures pinned together from packing material. My mind is thinking more in sensation, color, and form, stretching beyond mental ideas of what I am looking at.

I'm taking an independent study in the pottery studio of the community college. After a long day of clinical work, I'm standing on top of a large heavy table, punching and ripping angrily at the clay at my feet. My feelings are volatile and burning. Doing therapy with a very young child who's been unspeakably abused has bruised my neutrality. My feelings cascade from the chaotic rage in my heart, through my hands, and into the clay at my feet. I'm not forgiving in this moment. A trio of faces is gradually forming: anguish, rage, and Buddha calm. I have a vision of putting them together as one. The clay is a receptacle for hard, unspoken feelings for the child, for my humanity, for the need to maintain neutrality and clarity in being with her and her hurt family.

Just now I alternately work on forming the faces of rage and anguish. Each is contorted, filled with intensity, frenzy. I'm in a space of my own, unaware of anyone or the studio. A voice accosts my brooding, and I pull my face around to the sound. A young, sweet-faced student looks up at me, disbelief and curiosity in her eyes,

"Are these really your feelings?"

I look down toward her as if miles of ether wobble the air between us. I can't speak anything to her chaste look. She knows nothing about such grief, and I have no way in the vast distance between us, and in the bedlam in my heart, to tell her anything in words just now.

I want to hang the trio on the wall in my office, but I've made the clay too thick, bulky. It won't hang anywhere, even on the side of my garage. I find a place for it in the bottom of my garden, hidden under a bushy, red-twig dogwood.

Leigh and I take many classes together, enormously enjoying each other's zest in quietly rowdying up students and teachers. We are having a quiet tea together one Saturday in my apartment. Nothing is ever quiet with Leigh, and we get high on enthusiasm. Suddenly I say, "You paint one way, and I, totally differently. What do you think what would happen if we painted together on the same piece of paper—an experiment?"

"Awesome!" she says. "But not at the same time. You start one, give it to me, we'll go back and forth with it, and see what happens."

I start in my studio with a swash blue-scarlet color, an arc on large, rough, half-elephant size watercolor paper, a starting gesture. I hand it off to her and wait. In her studio she adds a jaunty house and a long, fragile ladder up the side. I add, she adds, and we pass it back and forth in a dance with it. She uses contained symbols: arrows, stop signs, house forms, and ladders. I use brash gestural strokes with my abstracted bits of flower forms.

I get mad when she paints over everything I've done. Her painting is like archeology, layers and layers heaped on one another. I want fresh bits of paper left.

The colors in the paintings we make are bright, in motion, alive. A white tower sits at a precarious angle in a swirl of black, green, and red. Its top is crowned in golden yellows with arcs of white and black arrows whizzing around it. A fragile outline of a tall, skinny house looms through black clouds at the side.

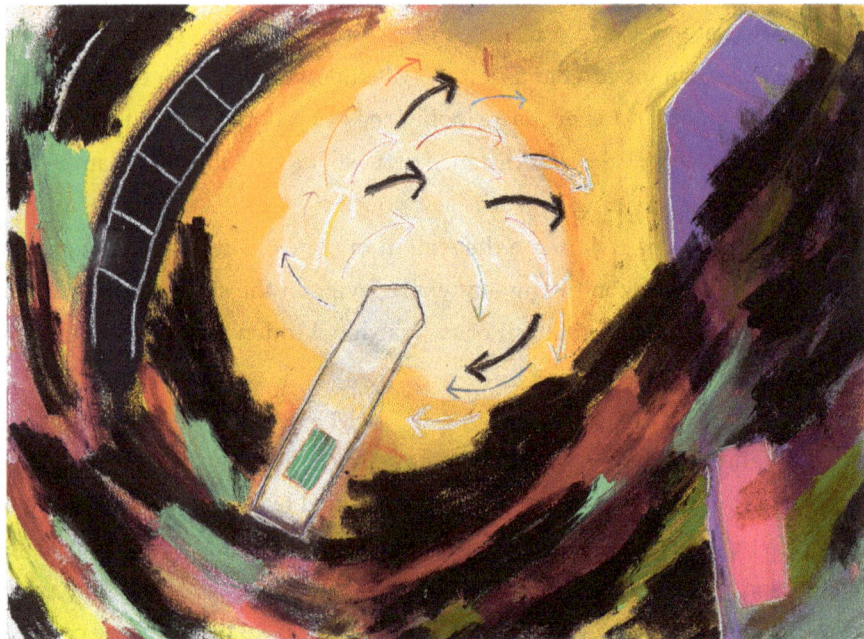

Death is a conscious part of these paintings. Death lives inside both of our lives, present, vibrant, and vital.

After we have made many paintings together, again on impulse, we push-pin a two-by-two group of paintings onto my white high-ceilinged living room wall and see them become a single mosaic. We add more around them so they fill up the whole wall, twenty-four paintings. The effect is a swirl of color and motion, each piece radiating energy to the others. It is a deep, wild expression of the life of life, death inside it.

A sweet little 1906 cottage is for sale in town where I work. I'm anxious about it because I haven't bought a house by myself. Leigh urges me past my reticence, advocating for the much larger studio space there for me. There are still exterior shingles hanging on one wall of this add-on room, a skylight, and French doors opening onto the back porch. It's an odd addition, and lovely for a studio.

George and I had bought our first house on the edge of Brooklyn Heights with a tiny inheritance from my father when our daughter was born. It was right across the street from the apartment house we lived in. It was an 1850's Greek Revival townhouse that had been a rooming house for decades. We spent weeks with crowbars and sledge-hammers bashing out drywall partitions. The contractor objected, but we moved into the bottom floor early in the renovation anyway, making him install a toilet and hook up all the house's electricity to run five appliances in place of a kitchen. For weeks I washed dishes in the bathtub. Between nursing the baby, I ran up a twelve-foot ladder in the parlor to spackle the ceiling or to create patches to the Greek classic plaster moldings. Learning how to repair them was my special project, and I took pride in my solutions. Then we painted everything linen white around the magnificent high windows. The house seemed to shrug off its decaying years and stand taller in the majesty of its earlier plan.

Buying this cottage now is possible with a little inheritance from my mother. So many years later in my life, she is giving me grounding and sweetness in this house. It has two large mullioned windows in front, with two magnificent Douglas firs standing in front of them, making the house feel secluded by woods. Window boxes with flowers and a stone path to the door decorate it like it is a cottage made for Goldilocks and me.

It is older than the houses around, its been vacant for a decade. I'm curious about its older story and find historic real estate maps and city directories in the history section of the library. A young carpenter got a promotion in 1905 to head carpenter in a major building firm in town. The following year he built his own house, his way, out in a meadow, edging on a long ravine of woods out of town.

I like this picture of the man making his own way; I sense his enthusiasm poured into the walls and floors of this house. I realize that I, too, am a new person in this house. I'm like a lizard who's lost a foot and grown another. I lost speech and grew feelers waving in the air.

In the center of the studio I construct a large table from two outsized doors, place them on sawhorses. More space makes it possible for me to work larger. I love rough, heavy, thick paper, but the double elephant paper I'm thinking about is expensive and too large to store easily. I buy pieces of canvas and try using it like the coarse watercolor paper, wetting it as I would paper. I paint with rags, not brushes, spreading and smearing color into the wet, selectively taking up some of the color with towels as it begins to dry, rewetting, and taking up color again. This works.

A local tent and awning company carries art-quality canvas, cheaply, and I buy a whole roll of it. I rip six-by-five-foot pieces, don't stretch them, and then hang what I like with tent grommets.

I expand the painting surface dramatically, and with it the passion. I paint from the scathing fatigue always in my body, letting it flow through my arms and fingers into the rags. Fatigue courses along through the paint and across the rough fabric and becomes passion to the eye. I start a piece with a germinal idea, and it moves on its own across the canvas. My hands follow the fatigue from my body into the form.

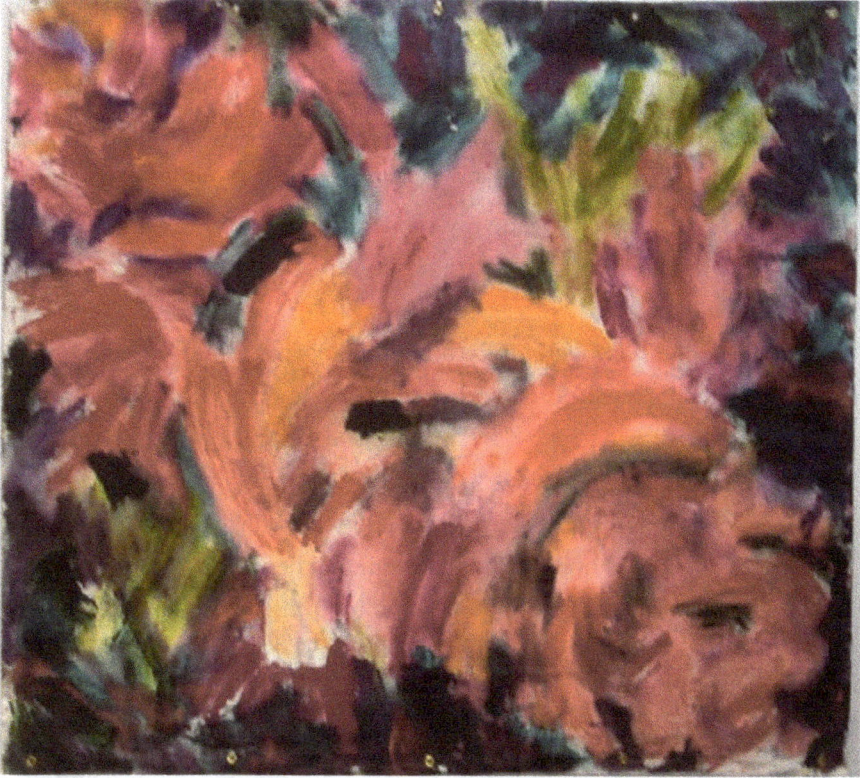

Abstract rose forms run diagonally down a canvas in blue-reds and red-oranges with flairs of green and yellow. Tree forms emerge, and I begin making large abstract faces of women inside the abstractions.

I'm more willing now to experience the daily soft presence of death that lives in my brain. The paintings dwell in an ecstatic place of living and dying all at once. There is messiness in the utter beauty of the two weaving in my life. There is no paradox. I'm conscious of living a huge "Yes" to life and of walking with death as an intimate at the same time.

This period in the Pacific Northwest is one of bold reconstruction in my life. The environment and the culture are easier for me here, and I expand my physical, professional, and art worlds to encompass more work, more pleasure. But my aphasia is still the center challenge in whatever I do. I have to streamline my life as Dr. Sarno taught me in the beginning. Choosing mindfully is essential even now, ten years after the stroke. Overwrought fatigue is still a hazard, and there are days lost to it.

I make remodels to this house, tear plaster to studs. The bathroom is deep brown marble. I try to imagine it as a mossy cave, a stone bathing grotto, but the old stains invade my sensibility. Instead I make a white tile bathroom with white linen shower curtains, and very much want to ask my friends to tea there.

The kitchen has two closely adjacent doorways. One used to be an entrance from the back porch and now opens to the short hallway to my studio added to the back of the house. The other is from the kitchen into the dining space. The doorways, side by side, are archaic; the caprice of the layout undermines any small order I so lately have in a kitchen. I consult a New York colleague who lives her spare time in her kitchen.

"Tell me how to think about designing a kitchen! I can't believe the glitz of the mags."

She draws out three activity maps for me, showing me how they work functionally. I choose one that fits my disordered mind and the actual space I have. Tearing plaster to studs again, I put in track lighting, white counters, a new stove, open shelves for dishes and cookware I can see, a standing cabinet for hiding groceries. I put down oak flooring in the kitchen and into the dining area to match the living room. I still have appalling trouble following a recipe and sequencing the whole plan from shopping to making, but my body is at ease in this new kitchen. I can see things I need around me. This kitchen helps me move from one activity to another more smoothly. It frees my mind from its struggle for organization.

I delight in discovering the archeology of this house as I make changes. I find an old front doorsill in an odd place, across the house. There are paneled walls beneath the plaster of the bathroom, next to the old doorsill. I guess that the paneled walls were the original entryway, maybe a mudroom. I find a long boarded-up window in the kitchen. I imagine the original face of the house when it looked from the side in a different direction across fields. The back of the carpenter's house had a long porch that faced into the deep wooded ravine. I see that it was a lovely place to sit in the evening looking into the trees, hearing the birds after the hard work of the day. Now my neighbor's house sits where those woods were, the ravine filled in decades ago.

Underneath the strata of change I see the house he built. I feel the layered presence of this home. The sensing is like the Brooklyn townhouse. This time I am deepening further into the intention and the sentience of this house.

As I rest so much of the time in this house, I feel kindness in the way light falls softly across the angles of the walls, peacefulness in the peaked shape of my bedroom in the attic. There is airiness as I walk in the upstairs hallway and light from the gabled roof and windows that were added there.

The house has a comfortable, old, lived-in feeling and is gentle for my body. As I live here I feel its energy of homey gracious¬ness supporting the simplicity of my own living. On days when my body aches for silence and rest, I feel the house softly close around me. It has a physicality of ease and seems to have a language for me of silence, space, and containment.

As my physical, work, and art worlds expand, so my sensory awareness to my environment gets bigger. I begin to see and feel more and more the life force around me, more perceptive to the sentience I have never before seen and to the sensory languages I've never heard.

I'm agitated by the expanse of rough, patchy grass in the odd shaped yard jutting from the back of the house, irritated by lack of the wild or beautiful. Five trees hunker at the edges, a beautiful ornamental cherry tree, an ancient plum, and a double blooming dogwood. It is an early spring afternoon. I sit on the back porch with my daughter, who's visiting. We sip tea and gaze out at the scrappy expanse. I tell her I'm at a loss what to do with the yard. She thinks for a moment then suggests a vision to make a luscious urban forest. Struck with this idea, I find a landscaper who thinks like a poet in patterns of green and likes this unusual opportunity to make such a plan.

He sledges the concrete basketball practice court at the bottom of the yard into pieces and fashions two beautiful little terraces up the sloping yard. He makes one of them border a quiet glade at the bottom. Red-twig dogwood circles part of it at the base of the dogwood tree. On the other side he puts five wild rose bushes on top of the terrace and makes a graveled center. It becomes a meditative center, and I place a small iron table and two chairs there.

Around the other terrace further up the yard he plants myrtle, an odd shaped pine tree, and several small madronas near the cherry tree. Black gravel paths make contrast with the many greens, and yes, he leaves a small lawn for me by the back porch for sitting and picnicking. An open circle at the center of the yard, carpeted with blue star creeper, becomes a place for stones, a small ceramic pool with a few water plants, and a little garden deity.

Another spring afternoon, perhaps a year after the garden has begun to settle into itself, I'm kneeling, weeding around the myrtle. At the same time I watch two crows who often sit on the telephone line running through the alley. One has a leg bent back at a right angle, so he stands on his shin. He is agile and balanced all the same; so it seems he has lived this way a long time. I say "he" because I watch him loving her. Sitting at the end of the wire near the street, he looks casually at her and sidles slowly down the wire, moving closer and closer to her at the pole a distance way. It is a little dance, or the flirtation of an old steady couple. He could just fly to her, but he doesn't. I watch her, sitting at the far pole, seeing him come to her out of the corner of her eye. She doesn't move. He edges up to her and nestles beside her, and she snuggles against him as he grooms her tenderly.

None of the crows in the nearby tree colonies ever come to sit this wire, so I think the two are patriarch and matriarch. This is their domain. Eventually, he notices me watching and comes to sit on the garage roof across from me as I sit on my porch with my morning coffee. I'm in East Coast intellectual mind, and I observe him as I did the babies in my research nursery, curious, without theory.

When I stepped into the small world of baby research as a new Ph.D., I wanted to explore the mind of the baby. I wanted to learn how a baby thinks and knows before words, what affects it. I wished to carve down through the silt and rock layers of time to witness the unknown below the surface of adulthood.

Babies are great watchers. They delight in observing through all their senses the many levels of the world around them, comparing and organizing all of it. They do this without words. Receptive to language, they experience and organize the world not in words, but rather from all the sensory perceptual modes they begin with.

When my daughter was just a few months old, she watched the patterns of light and shadow cast on the wall in the living room where she sat, the light coming through the Venetian blinds. Later in the day when the patterns changed to a different wall, she found them there, always gazing with absorbed interest. A couple of months later I played Hayden's Toy Symphony on our hi-fi. She listened carefully, bubbling with laughter whenever the toy instruments in the score were played. I played a lot of music for myself, but I played the Hayden especially for her because of the toys. It was she herself who appreciated the musical joke.

As a youngster I remember my parents taking me down the nighttime stairs, sitting me on a stool by the yellow and black enamel stove. They put newspaper over my head, making a tent for me to breathe the medicine water boiling in the brown cake pan. At two I had asthma, called croup then. I felt their concern for me, but under that sensed the uncertainties between them. In my wheezing lungs, tense and troubled, I knew their discontent, their grief. It was the newspaper that was telling, a curt, crisp reality, not a soft, enfolding towel.

Babies in the early months are lively in sensing their world with their whole bodies, collecting a multitude of information not yet encoded in words. Before a verbal mind develops, there is a sensing body.

My observing was not sweet and light in my early years. Not easily verbal, my sensory mind still held understanding of some non-verbal essence of what I experienced. I made my own sensory sense of my father and mother's worlds that held a core of me together. Then later it became a pleasure in my world to observe the immense variety in motion around me, the light and the dark, the sensory interplay.

Now with the constant struggle to find and cobble together words, the sensory and the non-verbal world around me is refreshing and intriguing — first sensing the house, and now the crow that flies over from his perch to sit on the peak of my garage. I observe him while drinking my morning coffee on my back porch. He doesn't just randomly fly in and out. He seems deliberate in his coming and his presence feels companionable. No words needed. His mate sits quietly on another roof at the edge of the yard, watching us. I watch his comings and goings, his activities tending her, flying back and forth to the huge crow families living noisily in nearby fir trees.

I find a flat stone one morning and place it near the bowl of water plants by the upper concrete terrace. It makes a place to leave pieces of bread for him. The first day he takes one piece, flies off with it down the alley, and doesn't come back. After a week he takes two, carefully holding both of them at once in his beak, the second one, I think, for his mate. Still he doesn't return for more. This is striking to me because crows are unabashed and gluttonous food gatherers. He makes taking the bread from me a more delicate act. It feels like a communion rather than a meal.

My critical East Coast attitude supports the continual natural observation of the crow and his mate. Such observations were what I did and taught in my baby nursery: watching, articulating and recording the details of behavior and relationship, allowing theory to evolve from observation, not placing theory first. My developing relationship with the crow is sweet and tender, crow and woman, living as neighbors. There is a non-verbal, non-mental language between us, interest and even affection across our large species differences. This non-verbal, sensory relating to another being is intriguing and curiously satisfying for me.

The two Douglas firs cloister the front of my house. A branch of one brushes my head, no matter how I prune it back, as I walk across the little stone path in the grass to my door. As I set aside the verbal and allow myself to sense into the sensory world around me, the crow and now the trees seem to make relationship with me. I step across the stones to my door this dusky evening and sweep the soft fir needles from my hair. I can think whatever I want about this being only in my imagination, but the sensation in my body is of receiving. It is like having the attention of a wise elder that I haven't asked for but nonetheless get. When my body, not my mind, responds with "Yes, thank you!" to the fir, there is pleasure, some new delight received. I have no mind logic for this.

One of the firs drops all of her limbs in a terrible ice storm. Many hundreds of trees in my neighborhood have simply toppled over with the great weight of ice. But this one does not fall on my house, which is so near it, but rather drops all of her branches, leaving a naked pole. I am relieved, but also touched by this. I know in my cognitive mind that the fir did not act with intention, but still, so many trees have simply fallen, on cars, telephone lines, houses.

In the night I set out little candles around her, make snow caves for them against the wind. They blow out, and I light them again and again. I wonder what the neighbors think, but I am unaccountably sad. My house feels naked without her presence.

A week later I sit in meditation with my drum, quietly sounding. As I painted my way though the verbal intensity of many Robert Bly conferences, I also learned a bit of drumming. It is now my private way of bringing in the New Year, to drum from ten to one or two, until sleep comes and falls into my bones. At nine I call Jake in New York, and she holds the phone out her window for me to hear the harbor boats come alive there with their midnight voices of jubilation.

The New Year is coming. Deep into the drum, I feel into the turning of the cosmos. I notice the damaged fir tree slip into my meditation, and feel sensations of her trunk surrounding me, as though to enfold me. I do not understand this, but I feel gratitude from her, feel her strong trunk surround my body. Against my ordinary judgments, I feel a relationship with this tree, as if in her dying she is offering protection to me. My life feels more settled now away from the turbulence of New York City, but the thought is not far of other health dangers and death under my skin.

I feel some larger, non-verbal truth here for me. Like the tree, I am stripped of the branches of my speech. I remember the grace of her branches leaning down to caress my face as I come into my house. I remember, too, a boulder in the middle of some Oregon woods where I stopped for a moment, breathless from running. I leaned heavily against the stone, and I hear a story from it of rushing water and the force of an ancient glacier that pushed it far from home. I am not asking for this, but the world around me seems to be talking, relating to me. In giving up so much of my verbal self, the sensory right side of my brain seems to listen to non-ordinary sensory communication.

It is a cooling, blustery day in the fall and I am in the center of my yard, pleased by some of the blue star creeper still in bloom. I look up at the crow standing on the telephone wire and notice he's a little unbalanced there, not his usual sturdy stance. His sleek midnight coat is different—disheveled, feathers ragged, grayish. His mate is grooming him carefully now, not the other way around. I think he isn't well.

This year's winter is particularly harsh and cold; I worry about him absently. Early in February I see him poking around in my front yard. Unusual to see him there. Nonetheless, I'm glad to see him; he's made it through the winter!

Then I don't see him again, stretching into weeks. One early spring morning I'm sitting on my back porch with my coffee. Six black silent crows fly into the barely budding cherry tree near me. I've never seen crows there. They perch in a stark even row, at attention, stand there without a sound. My breath catches sharply with the magnitude of their presence. Then the six silently fly off in deliberate unison. My heart stops in my chest, for then

I know that my old friend is dead. I try to think otherwise, but it is no use. I cannot rationalize this.

A year later I'm telling an old college buddy the story of my crow friend. We're sitting at the iron table in the little sunny glade in the bottom of my yard, now a burgeoning a young forest of red twig dogwood bushes around us. Suddenly around our heads a wild cacophony of crows circles, and we can barely hear each other. I struggle to go on with the story as they continue their chorus around it. When I'm done, they abruptly stop, as if the crows have punctuated my story with theirs.

A few years later I've remodeled the garage into a garden office with windows facing out into the yard. Ruth Chaffee, my professional colleague, and I are having an afternoon peer session, talking together about more difficult concerns in our work with patients. We're chatting first. I've gone to my son-in-law's recent talk at a bookstore in a nearby city. I'm thrilled with what a wonderful storyteller he is, and I begin to relate to her part of the story he told about the great mystic Rabbi, the Bal Shem Tov.

Before I know it I tell the whole story:

An old peasant farmer had for many years promised himself he would take the long journey to pray with the Bal Shem Tov at Yom Kippur, the deepest day of self-reflection for the new year. He began to walk, with no goat to ride and no passers-by to give him a lift. After many days he was still far away, and now he was in the dark forest night. A simple man, he didn't know the prayers, but did know the Hebrew alphabet. He called to God, "You know all the prayers; please arrange these letters into prayers," and all night long he repeated the letters.

A great cacophony of crows whirls and caws above my garden, intruding their loud voices into my telling.

The letters formed themselves into birds in protection of him, but he missed Yom Kippur by three days. He came into the synagogue feeling foolish, but the Bal Shem greeted him generously, "We have been waiting for you! Because of you, all of our prayers were answered. It is the Sabbath and you will feast as my honored guest."

I finish the story; the crows are suddenly quiet and leave. There is no reasoning for it. I listen and watch.

Living by myself is a haven. In this home that I have shaped for myself, I have silence, a lazy sparkling stream that meanders softly through the banks of my brain. Solitude is also here, allowing me to sit at the silence stream for reckless amounts of time, careless of need for company. In my clinical work my driven brain searches for words, rushes on at flood stage, heedless to stop. Silence, solitude, and music eddy through my brain, handing over the torrent to rest.

I am not lonely in this haven, but I am alone in this house. I want a non-talking companion who can share both the house and the haven with me.

The white standard poodle is standing in the doorway of the cramped office where I am sitting at the dog shelter. Her body hangs limp from her spine, her head droops, eyes stare at the floor. My heart aches for her already. She is not going to move into the room or toward me on her own.

I've not had a dog for decades. I felt daunted with the thought, until I fell into the bottomless brown eyes of a white coiffed Samoyed standing in the courtyard outside a dog show. His eyes mesmerized. His whole body vibrated with alertness, intelligence. He took in everything around him! That's the kind of dog for me, I thought. The standard poodle is my choice, also smart and loyal, but hair not fur, no shedding, hence no allergy for me.

I've arrived at the shelter after Poodle Rescue, the breed clearinghouse, called this morning. "I have the perfect dog for you, but you have get her now! She is regal, acts haughty, as if she knows she's in the wrong place."

I've hastily rearranged my schedule, and now I'm wedged against a clutter of drab little desks, signing adoption papers for this poodle whose life is unknown to me. She is brought to me. There is no happy tail-wagging, oh-take-me-home-with-you attitude. She is clearly sad and, I think, uncertain about what is next. We will have to warm to each other. Awkward is the note as we take an initial walk together under the trees in the fenced exercise yard. She stumbles around her feet, as though she has lost how to use them. Her dazed mood is contagious, and I, too, am unbalanced, inept to put her at ease. We don't get into rhythm. I think, maybe they won't let me take her.

However, in the car she sits pert in the front seat. I'm talking to her, telling her I wish I knew her name. Sally comes to mind. I cast that aside, thinking I can't possibly know that. Anyway, she doesn't feel like a Sally to me, too silly and common. I see a more majestic spirit underneath the lost dog. I tell her I will call her Sahaya, a name from Sanskrit especially for her. It means beautiful companion.

On the way home I stop off at a groomer, fancying that a bath will wash off some of the effects of her trauma. She emerges taller in her white loveliness and looks me in the eyes for the first time. While I wait for her, I buy a pretty blue leash and collar and put them on her.

In front of my house she steps lightly out of the car onto the grass and looks carefully over at the waiting open door. She pauses. In a sudden movement she slips out of the new collar and tears off down the sidewalk. I'm holding the slack leash in my hands as I watch her white fluffy tail vanish in the distance.

I pull myself out of shock, close the open front door, and run after her. Looking down each street I hope to see her tail swishing in the air. Nothing. I cross a busy street into the nearby university campus, thinking, could she have gotten across this street? I imagine her limp body smashed against the grill of an oncoming car. My body flushes hot with fear.

Then I spot her at the top of a grassy rise, lying there watching me through the grass. "Sahaya!" I call out, happy to see her face. As I come near, she runs away, and stops a distance away, waits and watches. I come near, and again she runs off and waits. I'm befuddled by this run-off-and-wait game, scared in my bones that she'll just run away. I imagine both Poodle Rescue and the shelter saying, "You lost her after only TWO HOURS?!"

I can't think of a better plan, so I keep tracking. She peeks around the edge of a building at me. I'll be cagey, I think, and creep around behind her and surprise her. When I get there, she has run behind me to the other end to eye me. I shout to some students. "Catch the dog! Catch the dog!" She lets them get close, but then nimbly steps around them, and they go off, not staying to help.

I feel like a cat being tantalized and tricked by a mouse. She knows the meaning of this game. I don't. I think maybe she is waiting to see if I will get mad. It is a test I have to pass.

Struggling with fear, I see a campus security guard and throw my desperation at his feet. He's amused, but takes up the challenge, laughing. We make a plan to form a triangle between her and us and then close in on her. At first she slips around us with ease. Then we move into synchrony when she runs into a bin of woodchips. She's cornered. Gasping for breath from running, I walk slowly toward her and struggle to talk softly. She looks up into my face with a tender look in her eyes. It is a gentle moment, and she doesn't move to bolt. I say quietly, "Let's go home and have some dinner… You must be hungry."

I put the collar on, more tightly this time. Her body relaxes. We walk in an easy cadence together the four blocks back to her new home. I have passed the test. Through this wild run around the campus, she's made the choice to be with me.

She won't let me out of her sight now, but she cowers when I raise my voice even slightly. I walk behind her, and she jumps away, startled. She has been hit and yelled at, I think. Although she is seven years old, she isn't spayed. Perhaps she was a puppy mill mother, a commodity, physically cared for, but severely treated. That owner didn't see her willingness, her gentle, lovely spirit.

I take her everywhere I go. In the hardware store a little fluff of a dog a quarter her size stands in front of her with eager face and wagging body. Sahaya stands like a frozen statue. I lean down close to her ear and whisper, "It is OK. That dog wants to be friends with you." I stroke her back, and her body softens.

I take her to a dog daycare, and a couple of days a week she slowly warms into having dog friends. They cluster around when she comes, and she, in her sweetness, becomes a favorite playmate. When I come to get her,

her whole body wiggles, her eyes shining. She is like a little kid saying, "Hey Mom, I had a great time!"

One day I leave my lunch on the kitchen counter and go out of the room. She seizes the moment and steals my lunch of triple crème cheese and French bread. I come back to crumbs on the floor and a dog licking up the last. She hunches her body down and looks up at me through her hair, trembling. She wonders what I will do to her. Despite losing my fine lunch, I'm euphoric she's willing to make mischief. I nuzzle her, and she presses her body against me. She pulls her head back, looking eye to eye with me as if to say, "I didn't expect this!"

Finally, she acts like an ordinary dog with me. But she is anything but ordinary.

I've been studying a Seik/Tibetan healing meditation practice, and Sahaya comes with me, sleeping by me for the whole day. She seems content to soak in the healing aura of the room every time we go. For me the practice soothes my verbal mind with its directed meditative wordlessness. After few months she leaves my side, carefully walks around people lying on mats as client or sitting as healer. In the practice the healer lays hands lightly on the client to sense them in meditation. Sahaya is deliberate not to step on anyone, then chooses someone and lays her body against them. She continues to do this. They tell me she is a comfort and help. Watching her, I am impressed by her sensitivity to the humans around her and her intentionality in making choices. The meditation healing practice is wordless, sensory, without preconceptions. She can do that, perhaps more easily than I. Her presence in my life is taking me deeper into the sensory world around me, another non-verbal relationship, this time an animal showing empathy, sensitivity, discernment, and intentionality.

She goes with me to my office, content to sit by my rocking chair at first, but soon, wagging her whole body, she becomes the greeter at my door to each patient. One day in a session with a troubled patient, she gets up, sits facing me, and puts a paw on my arm. She wants something. "What?"

I ask myself. It's not food. It's not pee-pee. I don't know. I pay her no more attention. She sits back for a moment, watches me, puts the paw back on my arm, and leans her face directly into mine. "OK," I say to her.

I have a thought that she wants me to do something with the patient. I don't know why I think this, but I head more plainly into the patient's worries, and the patient responds, finding a pathway through her sense of helplessness today. Sahaya lies back down and goes to sleep. I notice what Sayaha has done, but I don't give it credence until it happens again ... and then again. She gets in my face, and if I change what I am doing, I do better work and she lies down content.

Another day a session is about to end, and Sahaya rushes to a side window, jumps up, paws on the sill, body aquiver, making distressed, sighing sounds as she watches the next patient come through the gate and into the garden. She leaps across the room, sits with her nose to the door as though looking through it into the waiting room. She is oblivious to me and the patient still in the room. She is all attention to the next patient coming into the waiting room.

When I meet the patient, she looks terrible: clothes in disarray, body shaking, struggling with tears. In the session Sahaya sits close to her, attentive, seeming to hang on her every word. She alternately nuzzles the woman and lies on top of her feet.

I'm amazed by who she has become and how narrow my own vision has been. I didn't know she could have such subtle discernment, empathy, and presence—beyond some humans I have known. She has put herself in relationship to me and my work, shows me what she is thinking, in fact, giving me advice. I see her immense language and it is clear. No words needed.

My brain is changing, becoming a different brain. Art is not only resting and balancing the left, verbal part of my brain; it is promoting and enlarging the right, creative, gestalt side. I live more in the right brain now, finding huge, unexpected, undreamed pleasures. I'm experimenting, creating variety, playing with all manner of art. I didn't grow up artistic, rather reluctant, even fearful. The sensory world is my playground now.

Still, with so much effort finding and expressing with words, pushing at higher and more intense levels of functioning, my mind and brain are also expanding boldly into the sensations of observation and vision. I have always been a phenomenologist, looking and wondering. My brain began recovering in New York with making art, visiting galleries and museums, looking as an artist at the cityscape, at people, at the wild variety of shapes and colors. Here in quieter surrounds, luxurious for a badgered brain, I sense more into the details of felt space, relationship, motion, and presence. My body is less under siege from fatigue and healthier away from commotion and the riot of stimulation. The physical exercise practices—flexibility, strength, and aerobics—I started in the Brooklyn club in the basement of the old St. George Hotel were first to de-stress the enormous buildup of fatigue from pushing the verbal so hard. Gradually, they began to create variety, strength, and pleasure in my body. A happy body better supports and partners a beleaguered brain. Here in the West, my body is more rested and open. It becomes more responsive to kinesthetic perception: sensations of movement in muscle, tendon and joints, muscle sense, and sense of body moving in larger space. Yoga is a practice for me to become more aware of all that array of body sensation.

In the soft, ancient environment of the Pacific Northwest and in my home, I rest into receiving the array of sensory sensation. Phenomenalism, without a clutter of verbal theory, observing for the sake of observation, finding what theory that evolves. Crow, Sahaya, my house, the firs, and landscapes have become intimates. My mind finds a kind of sentience in the sensory details of these relationships. My body, brain, and mind reach out to them, and surprisingly, they reach back. Sensory communication is evolving: between me and crow and the crow families that sing/caw my morning awake, between me and the spaces in my home, between me and silence. I'm experiencing new languages not given by words or sometimes even by communicative sounds. These non-verbal languages are sensory syntax, sensory language, felt though my body.

Babies do this naturally; they have a capacity to extend their abundant interest to almost anything novel, to expand their sensory experience. I'm standing in a hospital cafeteria at lunchtime. The five-month-old baby, arms waving, nearly leaps out of his mother's hold of him with a joyful expression on his face looking at a service dog. Babies also love looking at another baby, happy recognition, the beginnings of friendship.

Crow, dog, and house are doorways into companionship, into reciprocal awareness, a kind of sensory empathy, less cognitive. I'm seeing more of what my brain can do, what it is willing to do. I'm willing to dissolve conceptual boundaries of mind to see what can happen.

Without much engaging words or the left, damaged, limited side of my brain, my world is expanding. With these new encounters, my visual kinesthetic sensory systems and my right brain are moving into non-ordinary relationships and non-ordinary places. A brain has the capacity to move to other places, not just in imagination, rather to connect and move energetically into the surrounding world. Mystics do it, and spiritual adepts too.

I'm not particularly aware of these processes now, more quiet enjoyment, pleasure in detail, and connection with the world around me. These expansions become a platform for much larger non-ordinary experiences to come.

My daughter, her partner, and I sit huddled together, ears pressed against the Boston Acoustic speakers in my living room, the sun streaming over us in the late afternoon. With the static and roar of the turned-up bass, we're struggling to hear snips of the shaman's voice. "She told me it might not record," my daughter says lightly. "Her energy field interrupts the best recording systems."

There are so many things I don't understand. This is one. My daughter's health is deteriorating just as her career after graduate school is getting underway. Her medical treatments are at top dosages, her health is declining, and she has been told to stop working. She has diligently tried many alternatives in addition to conventional medicine to support her health. She consulted the Lakota shaman and has come to discuss it with me.

My daughter is a brilliant, remarkable, and sensitive young woman. "I see a glass ceiling above her that she hasn't, somehow, blossomed through," I think to myself. "There is more for her to be in this life." I wonder about some truth under the strange story the shaman told about a terrible limitation in some other life that affects her health now. She is limited by something she can't see despite her intelligence, insight—and willingness.

My daughter and I studied the Lakota Women's Medicine Wheel for four years with the shaman. In a rural lakeside home scented with smudge, we listened to the journey of the sun across the directions, going often into the lush yard to practice the teachings. I listened to the shaman explain the world of Native American spirituality, oneness with the natural world, and a native woman's way of relating to it. I saw her beautiful landscape in my cognitive mind. Even though I was then beginning to experience crow and poodle language and a sensory mind, I couldn't feel the oneness she taught. I couldn't learn it through her words.

My parents met when they were patent examiners and students in

Washington, D.C, he studying law, and she, physics and chemistry in night school. They married in the late '20s, Jew and Christian, radical for the time. Their families didn't quite shun them, but certainly didn't approve, not giving them the support that such a partnership would need then. After they parted in the early '40s, my mother journeyed through all possible Christian religious forms. I listened and saw, with curiosity. One of my father's sisters, a humanist, Zionist, Conservative Jew, took me under her wing, shared elegant Jewish family Friday night ceremony with me when I visited my father, gave me a sense of belonging to them, mentored my searching through letters.

There was no way I could choose one of these traditions over the other. In my bones I was both, neither, and all. Rebelling as an early teen, I stood up in front of the Methodist youth fellowship to complain about the lack in the church of real tolerance and respect for other religions. "I cannot think this way any more," I said, and walked straight from the room in a huff.

Much as my mother had done before, I went on a journey to find a better spiritual place for myself. I found the Unitarians, broad minded and intellectual. Agnostic, uncertain, most of my life, I waited for something else, much larger, more inclusive.

I'm still an East Coast agnostic despite the experiences I've had here in the Pacific Northwest. I can't fathom the story about another life a thousand years ago that could affect my daughter's health now. It is beyond me, outside anything I understand. I'm a mother hen covering the chick with her wings in protection. "Nobody is going to mess with my daughter in this life or any other!" I think to myself.

She is thirty-something; she will make up her own mind. If she sets herself to do the ceremony the shaman recommends, I will be there for her. My life, rocked by the stroke, has already loosened its tethers to the ordinary. I already walk in strange landscapes.

I speak to my daughter first, and then ask the shaman on the telephone, "Can I help?"

"A parent has never asked me this before," she replies in surprise. She is silent for a long moment, then says, "You can't come into Lakota ceremony lightheartedly like a tourist. A healing ceremony like this is a life-and-death matter. Big energies will be in play and we could all die... Of course," she adds, softening her voice, "my job is to see to it that doesn't happen..."

"I'm willing to do this," I say.

"Then you will be the West Gate," she replies. "You will have work to do to prepare. Prepare to meditate and stay alert for many hours. Take good care of yourself so you have strength and endurance."

For love of my daughter, I rush headlong into this uncertainty.

Meditation has been problematic for me. Many years ago, the '60s, I was attracted to Zen meditation. It was avant-garde, and I only did it in fits and starts because the cultural divide felt large to me. I didn't want that to be so, but it was. After the stroke I tried Transcendental Meditation, much less of a stretch by then in the '80s. I thought the practice would be helpful against the relentless word retrieval chatter in my mind. But when I sat in my office between patients and used the Sanskrit sound given me to focus on, the process of emptying my mind was so arduous that I fell asleep instead. That didn't seem to me to be the point of meditating, so I didn't continue.

I talk to Ruth Chaffee, my clinical colleague. We are having coffee late one afternoon in a small café in the neighborhood and I've already told her I want to talk her about the shaman's story about my daughter and to ask help for a meditation practice that my brain can assent to. We chat a bit about our practices and the pleasure of getting together. Before I can tell her about the shaman, I suddenly lose thought entirely and drift into some other realm about the story, no words. My mind slips into the center of an expansive white cloud, my mind adrift between the strange, invisible realm of the story and my ordinary thinking and life. It is only a few moments, but I feel a quantum sensory shift happening well beyond the experiences of non-language with crow, poodle, house, and landscape. The change is unclear and confusing at this moment. My mind returns to the café, to Ruth across from me. I labor to tell her the story in starts and stops, to convey feeling dazed. Friend, clinician, and mystic herself, she steps in to my puzzlement with experienced compassion, begins to help me to unravel the pieces.

I sit in Ruth's home one fall afternoon in a comfortable overstuffed chair in her dark paneled small den. She is starting a meditation practice with me, to teach me in the manner of David Spangler, her teacher. She tells me to close my eyes, asks me to imagine a garden, in the "inner theater" of my mind. I settle my body and mind into ease. Seeing the garden is easy. I see details, walk around a central lawn space, look at beds of flowers bordered by small rocks with tall shadowy trees along one side, observing, surveying. Ruth brings my attention to some mossy rock steps in a corner of the garden, and I walk down, down, and down. I'm in a quiet deep place in my mind, and notice that the verbal chatter sits at the surface, pleasantly distant. The meditation focuses on visual imagery, on the intent of what we are doing together. My mind and brain feel a serenity that happens when I am making art.

I begin yoga in the home of a couple who teach in tandem in their living room. I'm in pretty good shape from step, aerobic, and flexibility classes at the Family Y. Standing on a long purple mat in a meditative place, I'm looking out their wide windows through the winter naked trees toward the gray shoreline of Puget Sound. The woman speaks, and I turn my attention back to the room. The deliberate movements of my arms up into Tadasana, mountain pose, lifting my side body muscles and move into Utanasana, hinge forward, fold my torso down until my fingertips touch the floor. I hold and relax into the posture for a few breaths. With my hands flat on the floor, I step my feet back into Downward Dog, an inverted vee shape, hips high. The sensations in my body are different than any other exercises I've experienced. The woman comes by me, makes small adjustments, touches my arms, making my inner elbows to face one another. The change shifts everything in my shoulders and across my upper back. The Downward Dog is both difficult for me and relaxing, a paradox that my body likes. As the months go on, I'm learning a new kind of body awareness. This, coupled with holding postures for minutes at time, gives me more physical endurance.

Ruth tells me the importance of having spirit guides for information, for support, and for protection on the path and in the ceremony. A few years before in a ceremony during the Women's Medicine Wheel study with the shaman, I was given Eagle as a guide. I left that weekend afternoon barely able to drive my daughter to the train station. I couldn't focus on where I was going, made two wrong turns, got quite lost, made my daughter frantically angry and almost miss her train home. Eagle is a high spirit in the Lakota belief, and I just couldn't make the leap to having a relationship with such a spirit. I wanted a common animal and was envious of the woman who got Beaver.

Eagle felt too big for me to handle then, and something bigger was shifting in me that I couldn't begin to articulate, similar to the difficult but new shift I'm having now with Ruth and the ceremony. Spirit qualities come from actual animal behavior. An eagle is observant of everything on the ground and in the sky, macro- and microscopic eyes. If I'm going to work in the non-material realms of the ceremony, then the observer part of me wants a spirit who can move and see in larger, wider spaces than I can myself. I already have this guide, and the power and perspective of Eagle now feels right to me in this new journey. I have a little more confidence.

I wonder about other guides. My job at the West Gate, the shaman tells me, is to ward off dangers until she is ready for them in the ceremony. These perils are energies, but she can't tell me what specific form they will take in the ceremony itself.

I think of crow, my old friend in life, who is still very much alive in my memories, and the tender relationship we had. In Lakota belief the spirit of crow slips between the worlds, shape-shifting the rules of both earth and spirit and flying in mystical realms. As I slip between the world of language-based thought and the sensory world, I can feel that connection with my crow friend. In life he slipped deftly between my world and his, showing me a new way of relationship.

I'm drawn to the Hindu goddess, the Great Mother Kali. The story is told that the old gods lost their power against the two demons of great evil, Shambhu and Nishambhu. The gods conjured Kali, with their last collective strength, born out of Durga's head. Riding a buffalo, Kali raised armies out of herself, likenesses and powers of herself. Directing these armies to aspects of ego, she fiercely vanquished evil, cutting clean with discernment and compassion. I want the support of such strength and clarity, a guide quite outside any of the traditions I know, an outsider as I am, a critical onlooker to the events that will unfold in the ceremony.

I meditate every morning in my living room and ask for the presence of Crow, Eagle, and the Great Mother Kali. I feel a different sensation in my body as each comes as though each is saying, "Hello, I'm here." My body bows forward spontaneously when Kali comes, and my head shifts right and left as if visually scanning some horizon when Eagle comes.

Ruth meditates with me in the beginning to support the questions I have about the interior heart, the intention of the ceremony. The answers I get from the guides are often sensory, non-verbal, and sometimes visual answers. I have to learn how translate them into what I can understand. The shaman gives me exercises to experience other beings, like a tree, a stone, the sun. One day sitting in my garden, its exuberant profusion fills my senses. The morning is chilled, and I'm wearing a fuchsia polar fleece coat with a big hood. Still chilly, I close my eyes and ask to be in the sun. Instantly I'm there. I see around me convulsive boiling, but my skin is not burning, only warmed. I am myself, observing, and I am not me. I am the same as the sun, so fertile we could make anything. Particles expand and combine, come apart, explode, and recombine everywhere all at the same time, all in vivid yellows and oranges, other colors I've never seen.

I am deep in the sun when a buzzing commotion at my ear catches my attention. My body is profoundly still, so the startle is not enough to affect my meditation, only enough to change where my attention is. I ease my head around and come eye to eye with a tiny hummingbird. I gaze at this green beauty dancing in the air. Neither of us flinches in this long moment, hummer to human. I'm not a flower with honey, and she goes off. In these moments I've surrendered to other possibilities of living in this skin.

Going into meditations with Eagle, I practice being an eaglet, snuggle with the other little birds into the central bowl of the enormous nest that Eagle makes high in the crook of a sturdy tree. I'm soft and downy gray like the others, and we vie for the food, bits of rodent, fish, that mother eagle picks apart for us. In another meditation I'm a little older as an eaglet and scramble up the edge of the nest to balance and teeter on one of the large sticks there. I practice walking back and forth on the stick and then take the risk to hop over onto a branch of the tree, the first effort toward flying. Gaining strength and agility, I hop and then take short flights across the nest and around branches of the tree.

I fly many times with Eagle in meditation across large almost infinite space, practicing awareness in her way of seeing the smallest movement in the air and on the ground. Later she makes rapid swings around me to protect me, acting as a shield. In all of these different meditation experiences, I feel what it's like to live as an eagle. With the sun, Eagle, and others, I'm stepping into larger realities of ordinary and non-ordinary beings, expanding my capacity for visual and sensory experience.

Nonetheless my mind often runs around a maze of certainty and uncertainty, of prudence and risk. I lose track of what my reality is, can't find a map of where the intersections of the actualities are in the different realms. I worry about getting lost in deep pathways way off track. In a letter to my brother, Ernie, whom I've not seen in many years, I write a small sentence about being in spiritual distress. I intend nothing with this, but within the week he's on a plane crossing the continent to see me.

We sit across my dining table with afternoon light coming through the lace curtains at the French windows beside us. The light bathes his face with a gentleness I have not seen before.

"Some years ago," he tells me, "I was in anguish about my life. In the middle of the night … sitting on my bed … I was in agony … where to turn? I cried out, 'God! … God! Help!' …I didn't expect anything. I only spoke the words. And God answered! For a long time we talked together. And I was comforted.

"Afterwards, though, I was terribly unsure of what had happened. Was it real? Was it my imagination? Was I crazy? I went to my priest and told him everything. He called in specialists, who listened to me, and after careful deliberation they assured me it was real."

Ernie, electrical engineer and devout Episcopalian, and I, psychoanalytic psychologist and agnostic, have different views on almost everything. His particular eclectic and clear mind coming to me through the turbulence of our shared history paradoxically gives me confidence. His is a voice I want among my guides.

With Ruth I try out some meditations to step together into the time of the shaman's story telling of brutality, torture, dishonesty, and betrayal. We agree each in meditation to go into a market village, dressed in plain, shapeless, coarse dresses with aprons. We meditate at the same time and at the end will share the different experiences we had. In my meditation Ruth and I get into casual conversation with three women on the road. They are friendly, and one invites us to her home for tea. In a small little room, we are sitting together on rough, couch-like benches. I'm wearing leggings under my dress and thick cloth footwear. Part of this disguise falls off and one of my shoes appears instead, one of my own leather Mary Janes. Ruth notices, in my meditation, and tries to distract the conversation, to gloss the over the mishap, but I feel endangered. I worry if they see what has happened, they will see me an alien and a stranger. I could be in great jeopardy, see the possibility of jail and brutality. I step quickly out of the meditation. I feel there was some dark reality there that I should be afraid of. I will not try this kind of meditation again.

My task is to be good at what I do for the ceremony. If the danger I felt in that meditation is part of it, then the shaman will have to be the one to anchor it.

In another meditation one morning, I ask about managing my own safety. I've journeyed high in the galaxy. I'm sitting on a golden chair circling the earth, the sky around me black, the sun blazing behind me. I lean forward to gaze at the earth, immensely beautiful in its bright blues and greens. Part of the black sky around me becomes palpable, feels dangerous, climbs up my legs, but stops at my knees. I am not alarmed, and feel safe in this large perspective with the planet arrayed below me. Out of the meditation I know I'll be able to manage whatever danger comes to me in the ceremony.

I realize also my psychoanalytic perspective helps sturdy me, because I am not surprised or dismayed anymore by the possibilities of the darker sides of consciousness. In clinical practice I've done extensive deep work with patients with old abuses never before discussed, divorces and relationships full of rage or anger. Some things are not so new. I remember, too, that the shaman is the center of the ceremony and holds everything.

It's early evening and I'm lying face down on a massage table. The small second floor office is in an old frame house rearranged for five practitioners. I'm eager for this bodywork tonight; my day has been too full. The therapist begins rubbing my scalp and caressing my hair, instant calming, and I fall into a meditative doze. The welter of words melts away like butter. She moves down my right arm. I feel the sensation of crow feathers, my arm becomes a stretched-out crow wing, coal black and shimmering. She massages my back and my leg, and the right side of my body changes into black feathers and the gray of a crow. She moves over to the other side, and my arm becomes an eagle wing, with long brown wing feathers separated at the end like wing fingers, feeling the bones of flight. My left side becomes an eagle body, with my leg having the feathery trousers of the eagle ending at the ankles just above the yellow talons of feet.

I've been massage-sculpted as crow/eagle. My head remains as my own my white head; I exist as human, crow, and eagle in one, and maybe the white head is also that of a bald eagle. I'm drawn into their spirits, clothed in them, one with them, like family. I think I want confirmation from the shaman, but I don't need it. The deep sensations in my body are a reality for me. While my human body lies on the table, my eagle and crow bodies tell me of other actualities of being, of flight, of the experience of their lives, of shifting into oneness with them—body knowledge.

I have tree roots extending wide and deep into the earth, and branches that touch into the spaces between galaxies. I am a dogwood, a Douglas fir, sometimes redwood sequoia, my sisters. When I move to my mountain home and step into the yard, the sequoias greet me, and I feel an invitation to settle at their roots. Like with my crow friend and the poodle, I feel the sensory reciprocity of non-verbal, non-cognitive language with many beings other than humans.

Apart from talking to Leigh, my painting buddy, my brother, and my psychoanalytic colleague, I hold much private about this journey. I don't yet have the language to speak these experiences of sensing and being in other realms with non-ordinary, non-material presences. When I try, other people's ears go deaf like I'm speaking into an empty room.

As the months of practice go by, I am more confident but still often riddled with anxiety and doubt, and I settle on a desire to be in the healing room itself, to watch what they're doing with my daughter. When I express my desire to protect her in my morning meditation, I see an enormous tree with a large space between the roots that encloses the ceremony. I observe my daughter, the shaman, and her assistants are all safe inside, and I'm sitting on the ground outside. My ear is pressed to the thick trunk and I can hear everything inside. Later I find that the West Gate is the porch just outside the shaman's ceremony room, with open sliding doors to the warm July day, where I will, in fact, hear everything.

The shaman calls on the phone to tell me her husband has been in a construction accident, is going into surgery, and will need recovery time. She is apologetic, but has to reset the ceremony for two months later.

I'm in a fretful temper a few mornings later. "All this effort for what? Will all this have any effect on my daughter's health?"

I call for the presence of the Great Mother Kali and tell her, "If you will heal my daughter, I am yours." When my mood is better, I am shocked with what I have done. I think of Faust, who sold his soul to the Devil in Dante's story. Have I done that? What is the reality of my request? How far does this sensory mind go? I have learned to put protections—a discriminating mind—in place, but have I naively gone too far?

Dogwood blossoms flood around my head and shoulders. Their scent hugs into my breath. It is a magnificent day. I'm sitting on a great rock near Ruth in a Japanese garden, and we are meditating together. I hear her opulent words calling in the spirits of the directions. "Come to us, Spirit of the South, with your moist, verdant vitality, your boastful rush of growth. Come to us, Spirit of the West, your deep waters, your running of emotion through the setting sun. Spirit of the icy cold North, come to us with your expanse of mind through forests of mystery where Eagle lives. And now come to us, Spirit of the East, your first scarves of light, your fresh scents of morning dew across the budding fields." This time together marks my graduation. She has brought me to the time of the ceremony, and I'm ready.

Now it is a soft sunny day in the rural mountain home of the shaman, and I put several pillows on the porch floor, hang two of my paintings on the side of the house behind me, one of eagle and a self-portrait, both large and awesome canvases. The West Gate, one of the four directional protective gates, faces into the dappled green of dense trees and bushes. I brought stones, a quartz heart, and objects I've made, a gold helmet, not knowing their usefulness. I'm told I can't leave this spot for any reason at all. "Pee in your pants if you have to," the shaman said sternly.

The Keeper of the East Gate, an old friend and psychiatrist, has been in service to her in many ceremonies. We chat easily, and then he warns me. "The dangerous energies coming will feint first to the East Gate, where I am, and then come full bore to you at the West Gate. The Fire Keeper has seen this in his meditation." My body runs icy cold; I'm afraid. Before I can speak, a runner comes, "It is time. We're starting now!" she says.

I step onto the porch at the West Gate, apprehensive, then abruptly I'm in deep meditation. Without plan, I put on the soul mask I made in the Women's Medicine Wheel. Wearing it today depicts my soul name. I am nakedly vulnerable with it on, but also in my spirit's power, able to face to the dangers that will come.

My daughter has been meditating at the fire below and comes onto the porch to enter the ceremony room. As she passes I can barely nod to her for depth of altered state.

The ceremony begins.

I call my three spirit guides. A sensation of power whooshes in around me, and I gasp, astonished. I sense in my body the Great Mother Kali around me and in my inner mind see her vast armies arrayed in front of me to my left. The spirit of eagle circles above my head. Crow is close above my right shoulder, and sometimes sitting there.

While I call them today, as so many other days, I feel a deeper, definite choice they make to come, to stand, and to act alongside me. I fully make the quantum leap into a larger sensory mind, know them as beings, essences, acting with me in a larger universe that contains the ceremony.

At once I'm aware of something unfriendly coming toward me. In my mind's eye it is hidden in the trees just in front of me. Without thought I take the rose quartz heart from my meditations out of my pocket and extend it toward the trees in front of me, cradling it softly in my hands. In my mind I declare, "I am here. This is my daughter's heart. You will have to go through me, kill me, to get to it." I draw the stone back and place it on my heart.

My observing self asks, "What the hell are you doing? What kind of stagecraft is this, so dramatic!" My meditative mind answers, "Shut up! I'm busy!"

For four hours I sit at the West Gate in meditation, a kind of prayer, fulfilling what I was asked to do. Occasionally there are breaks, and I come out into the soft green day. Once when I re-enter I sense a connection with the North Gate against another dangerous intent that moves in the woods between us, serpentine. Without thought I put on the golden helmet I made from one of my meditations connecting Joan d'Arc with my French ancestry.

With the helmet, I have no fear; I'm at attention. I hear voices behind me in the ceremony room, listen to them singing as I continue in meditation. I do what my intuition tells me. My ordinary thinking, organizing mind isn't at play. I trust what is happening in me and around me. I don't know how it affects anything or anyone else. I am alone here with my guides.

The ceremony has its narrative; the shaman, the Fire Keeper, the Gates, the dog who chose to sit with the North Gate, and certainly my daughter, all have their personal stories about what occurred. There are many individual truths and there are larger truths. What I tell here is only my own small piece, what happened for me.

It is early evening, and the sun is still low in the sky when one of the shaman's assistants comes and quietly says, "The ceremony is over now. You can stand down!" Somehow, it all seemed easy.

The mountain air is serene and cool. The ceremonial materials have been taken away; my paintings, pillows, stones, helmet stowed in my car. A dinner table is set for my daughter and me on the porch, and dinner is brought to us. We are left together.

She is sitting across from me, but I see her as standing very tall above me, beautiful in the twilight. She is wearing new clothes after the ceremony, a long green print dress. A wide protective turban has been fashioned around her head, a print complementary to the dress. She is magnificent.

Stillness contrasts to the potency of what we have each been through. There are few words between us for any of it. I eat, thankful for these moments together with her, before the scurry of the long drive back to her partner, who is waiting for news of her safety.

A door has closed behind me.

The crow sitting with me at my morning coffee, the dog coming into my solitude, the house holding everything, landscapes and trees calling, speaking to me, and death sitting in my damaged brain, all these and the others taught me, in their separate ways, prepared me to walk into this day.

I stepped through the passage, and now I can scarcely breathe.

PART THREE:
THE PATH OF SURVIVAL

Two shady green mountain ridges crest my drive to the Pacific Coast to land at a gray clapboard apartment on the beach. Watching the twilight on the sand with the water in constant agitation and tasting the gray, salty air coming through the window, my body and spirit begin to ease. They need this pallid quiet to sort myself out.

Into the calm the next morning, the telephone's ring sharply intrudes. My daughter is apologetic, but must tell me terrible news of the sudden death of a young friend from the Bly conferences. Heart attack. Some years ago he told an amazing story of swimming at twilight in the Gulf of Mexico near his home. He swam often there and said the water was flat and warm, silky. As he stroked through the water, a shark gently came alongside him. They swam for a long time, side by side this way, at ease with each other. He said he felt friendship, and safe; it seemed natural. After a time the shark moved slowly off.

I remember my crow friend, the same ease, coming into my life. But my friend's courage floods over me now, his willingness to step across vast difference and fear simply to swim together. His spirit is stepping into a larger vastness now.

Friends in New York City are coming together for him this afternoon. I want to resonate with them somehow across the continent. But I'm still in the after-aura of the ceremony and not ready. I take a long, creamy Jacuzzi soak in the beige-tiled bathroom. The steaming water creates a boundary and puts me into a hazy mind. My spirit is cleared by the hot baptism, and I'm ready. I put a few lunch things into a bag and take another for collecting. I set off down the sandy beach with not much thought for what I am going to do, some sort of ritual there on the water and beach.

A beachcomber, I see things as I go, a piece of driftwood looking much like a shark, then a dried starfish, crow feathers, a few wild daisies, some dry kelp, with a thought to make rattles later. All get put in my bag. I wonder what I am going to do, but nothing distinct comes to me.

The sandy beach turns rocky, and I keep walking. I'm wearing hiking shoes, and think I'm seeing actual little paths in the rocks for footing. I'm dreamy and walk right along toward a long rock peninsula as a destination, but I don't get to it. My attention is arrested by a tiny waterfall from high cliff that has risen on my right, ledges of crumbled rock. The water flows into a little pool in the rocks the size of my hand and drops down near my feet and disappears into a crevice. I'm entranced and fall further in reverie.

I haven't much experience making ritual myself, but it is my intention to make a good one now for my friend. I sit down on the ledge beside the pool of the waterfall to think, have my turkey sandwich and apple, but my mind isn't thinking much. Somehow it is full.

Finished with lunch, I cross the flat, brown-brown plateau of rock in front of me to a high promontory, where I watch the water spiraling far below. Still, I'm not thinking, yet a blessing begins to form. I take the driftwood shark from my cotton striped bag and cast it out into the air to watch it drop slowly down to the water. "Here," I say to my friend, "I give to you a watery companion and ally to swim with you on this new journey you are making ... whatever it is beyond where I am standing in this world. Your friend, shark, is a guide for you toward your next destination."

I send the crow feathers after the shark and speak about how crow is the spirit that flies between the worlds and a shape-shifter of the rules of each. "You, my friend, swam into the shark's friendship. You and the shark slipped between your different realities already in life. Crow, with shark, will help you move in this new immensity." I reach in the bag for the starfish, but it is no longer a dry skeleton. It has come alive again in the moist shadows. So it is right to return it to its watery home. As I send it into the air, "Be a starry beacon for my friend!" and I bless it for being willing to come with me to do this.

I stand for a while in this blessing dream for my friend, thinking and reflecting on the time I knew him. Finally I'm satisfied that it is finished. I turn from the water and toward the cliff behind me to return down the beach. My whole being is stunned. As far as I can see to either side of me, the whole face of the high shear cliff across from me is a gentle seeping waterfall.

An open temple appears to my inner mind on the flat rock plateau before me, scattered temple pillars, like ruins in Greece. I'm in a sacred place, and I wait. The Great Mother Kali speaks into my mind: "You have done well. You will serve in my temple." She has come, but there is no Faustian giving-up of my soul, no loss of identity I feared. She comes as part of the larger Mystery. She is the brave, strong qualities of a One God: constancy, clarity, justice, cutting very clean.

In the ceremony for my daughter I asked for the presence of my three guides. None has come to me spontaneously, except actual crows in the sky as reminders of my connection to their spirit. Seeing the temple spread before me and hearing her words, I feel deep blessing.

That the Great Mother Kali comes to me here this bright afternoon on this high promontory of rock affirms that my relationship with her is reciprocal and that the alliances with the other guides are also. This encounter with her is a reality to me.

When I lost speech language, I looked for non-verbal ways of relating, first art and music. Then I found non-verbal, sensory friendship with the crow, the poodle, became willing to sense non-ordinary relationships with trees, my house, the landscape, and to experience different realities in many meditations with the spirit guides. Finally in the ceremony for my daughter, I experienced Oneness in all things working with me, against me, and with the layers of larger relationships around the healing.

All of these encounters are part of a wide mystery. They are ordinary and extra-ordinary realities.

Another door has opened.

I've been on the sunny beach for more than three hours in the hottest part of a summer day, with no thought of sunscreen. I'm suddenly worried about that and move right along to my beach home. My feet swelter from the hot rocks. I get to the sandy beach and walk in the water, shoes and all, indulging in the wet, frosty water. When I return to my apartment, I'm as pale as when I left it.

There is no going back, even when I return to the ordinary world of my life. I experience the oneness of everything. At home at my breakfast table, I look out the window at a chickadee perched in the old plum tree there. The tree and the bird are distinctly themselves, but the chickadee and the plum are one with me here at my breakfast. We are diversity in the same life force. My spirit guides are also parts of the same oneness, except they are personal to me. The bird flies away to feast in another tree, while the plum tree sways in a gentle breeze dressed in the soft sunshine of the day.

Oneness now doesn't live in words in my mind. I can't understand any of it there. The verbal world insists on either/or thinking. While I participate in that world, I no longer live in it. Dualism and oneness are no longer a paradox. I can step out of dualism into oneness anytime I choose to notice.

As light is, I am both wave and particle.

I study with Ruth's teacher, David Spangler, for many years learning Western mystical practice. With him I expand my mystical perspectives further and learn a form of inner world service. A social activist in the '60s, I took to the streets of New York City with my baby to speak out for peace, nuclear restraint, and equality. Since the stroke in 1980, I haven't been able to be in such vibrant, noisy crowds; my body is too sensitive, a loss to my sense of justice and involvement in the world. With David I learn mystical techniques in which I can be proactive in planetary service while living with this body with its limitations, using its sensory relationships.

I lie on a narrow gurney in an angiogram x-ray lab, three monitors arrayed just above my face. I can see everything. The images of arteries and vessels on the screens are stunningly clear. Pointing, I ask the radiologist, "What's that! ...What's that! ... "

My speech has worsened rapidly over just a few months. I'm having a new cerebral angiogram to see what is wrong. Dye has been injected into my bloodstream to make the vessels visible on the x-ray plate.

I'm moved by what I see, nothing like the murky images I saw in the neurosur-geon's office so many years ago. The technology has advanced far. Clarity. No noise. What I see is amazing beauty, the trees of vessels and the patterns they make across the screens.

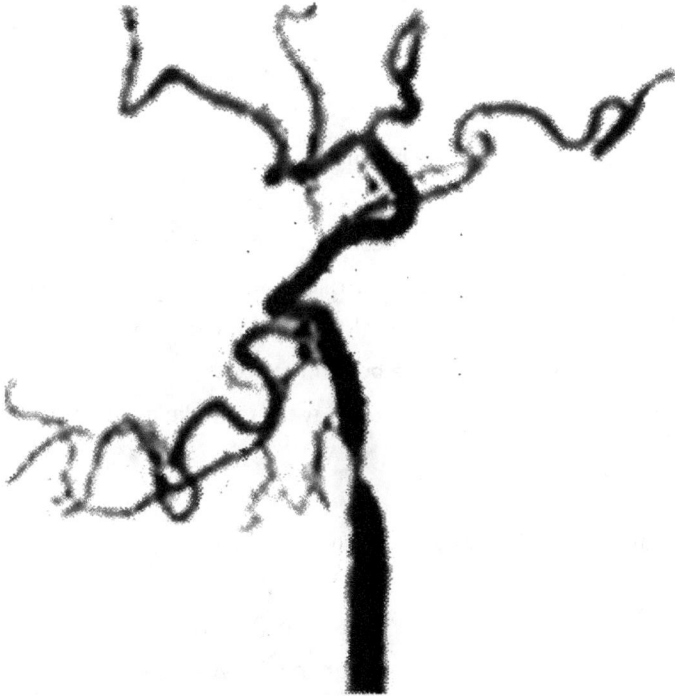

"You have to keep quiet!" The radiologist is stern. "I'm doing very delicate work here..." Mollifying me, he adds, "I will show you everything after I finish."

And he does.

The vessels have rearranged themselves in an extraordinary way across both my left and right brains in the twenty years since the surgery. Plaque slowly developed at the old surgical site, impeded the flow of blood, and restricted the expected expansion of the carotid branch placed in my speech brain. But many vessels from the right side and the back have, over the years, extended themselves widely into the left of my brain to offset the missing blood flow. The vessels and the life force of blood in them have moved into the empty places to cover the slack in the system for me. It is a visual story of renovation and reorganization.

I fall desperately in love with these images: brain arteries, staples, the place where the cut was made to remove a whole artery, decades ago. The vessels are delicate, strong, and vivid, magnificent in their enormous plasticity.

My damaged brains are beautiful.

They are breathtaking, these arteries, their flexibility to reconstruct themselves and the brain they nourish. They have been the bedrock of my rehabilitation, my ability to struggle to continue to do work I care about, and the creation of a whole new life beyond stroke.

I'm in love with these images. I want to make art using these rivers of life force.

Plaque at the old surgical site has all but closed off the artery feeding the verbal area of my brain. It is the reason my speech is faltering. An intervention radiologist a few months later goes into the artery again, does a cerebral angioplasty, reams out the plaque, opens the vessel, and puts in a little steel stent to discourage new plaque.

My daughter and her husband come to see me in the ICU, and smooth words fall out of my mouth. I'm giddy, laughing though my poor body is in cramps from lying flat the whole night. They have brought deli delicacies for lunch, and drop morsels into my mouth.

My desire to superimpose my cerebral vessels on self-portraits is stopped by technical difficulties. I'm a painter, and computer layering technology is beyond me. I experiment with sun prints in my backyard, sunlight through thick glass and x-ray film onto coated paper I make. The effect is a blueprint color, a vapid blue not nearly the bold impression I want. It isn't the vision.

Quite suddenly this easy speech changes again after a year and half. I notice that my speech becomes slower and I have more difficulty finding words. This goes on for weeks, more and more difficult. I'm alarmed with the steady decline I now see clearly. One morning I pick up the phone and call for an immediate appointment with my neurosurgeon. Leigh and her new husband come along with me to help me with language, so they can help explain for me, and to give me support. The neurosurgeon listens carefully to all of us and orders an immediate repeat cerebral angiogram. But I have to wait for two days to get on the schedule.

I'm frantic about the delay. I imagine terrible possibilities: I might collapse, have another stroke, get the wrong emergency care. I strew my house with Post-it notes hanging on strings: the front door, the arch between the living room and dining room, the kitchen, the studio, the stairway. I put doctor, hospital, and contact instructions on all of them.

Sahaya is so entwined with my life now, I walk around the house talking to her like a sister. "I'm going to the hospital to see what is wrong with me. Tomorrow I'll take you to daycare so you can be with your friends," I tell her. "Then you'll go to the kennel." I roll up her sleeping mat with one of my sweaty shirts and a few toys. The kennel is a spa for dogs. They pamper her outrageously, and she is happy there. I have no worry, only for myself.

I'm to go under anesthesia with the possibility that repair work will be done. I whisper into my daughter's soft shoulder, "I'm terrified this time!" The angiogram is normal, and the stent is working. The duty resident wants to discharge me. Groggy from anesthesia, I struggle to speak my hysteria. I can't leave without knowing what is wrong with me. I can't imagine the hour drive back and forth from one city to another, alone, for tests in the condition I am in. My daughter and her husband, and Leigh and her husband, argue relentlessly with the resident to have me admitted.

Five days of tests find no clear diagnosis, only a hypothesis that a medication I've taken before with no effect has now acted adversely. I've been complaining about pain in my head and shoulders; stopping the medication makes the pain subside. I'm optimistic because it isn't another stroke, but my body feels shaky and fragile and my mind struggles to come out of a fog.

"What happens when she can't live alone anymore?" my internist asks to my daughter and her husband. The three of us sit in a tight corner of the small examining room. Now he looks directly at me, "You all need to give some thought to that."

I'm bemused by the question. "It isn't time yet!" I tell my daughter later at home. "I have a life and practice here." Underneath the thin euphoria that it wasn't a stroke, I'm unsettled and can't see clearly. When they leave, I look forward to being alone for a few days and to the soft silence of the house.

The kennel is urgent. "Please! Sahaya really needs to be with you! She is doing poorly with us this time. She's not even eating the scrambled eggs and cheese we made special for her! We must bring her to you!" I'm weak, apprehensive, and look forward to seeing her anyway. I expect her to bound into the house, all wiggly-happy and relieved to see me.

She barely looks at me. Her body is limp and so transparent I think I can see through her. Her gaze is elsewhere, not here. I have a sinking feeling that she's thinking whether to stay in this life or go.

I wait a day for her to perk up, but she doesn't. I'm impaired enough that I won't drive. Friends take us to and from the vet. She is gravely ill with a rare blood disease. No reason. The vet gives a slim chance for her to live. I bank heavily on the chance, with high doses of steroids and soft baby food to entice her to eat.

Too weak to go up the stairs to sleep, she stays downstairs. I feel too frail to sleep downstairs to cuddle near her. She gains some stamina and labors to get up the four stairs to the first landing toward my room and lies there looking pleased with herself. Two days later she manages her way up the next nine steps to the second landing, lies there panting with the effort. I come out of my room one bright morning to find her all the way upstairs, lying in the hallway, wagging her tail as I come around the corner. With effort, she raises her head, looks at me, adoringly.

I am shameless, fall down beside her, hug her, in tears, full of admiration. "I think that you knew for a long time that I was not well, even before I knew myself. You had no way to tell me... You were heartbroken with worry when I was away so long."

As I speak, the words ring true. I think back on the many times she was accurate in responding to trouble in my patients, sensing the meditation students, walking around the room and choosing the person to be with. It is no stretch for me to think that she has been trying to help me all this time.

I'm moved by this dog and her devotion. In a sudden inspiration I tell her, "We will get training together so that you will have ways to tell me what you know. I will find someone to help us teach you to be a service dog for me... I adore you, and it's time to get you all the way well!"

We're downstairs together for the day and she sleeps there for the night. I come down the next morning, waiting for her little noises of getting up and moving to greet me with her eager face. The house feels empty; I don't hear her. "Sahaya!" I call. There is barren silence. I run out to the garden, expecting to find her there, but there is only stillness. My eyes scan the yard until I see her white back serenely stretched out on the ground near the porch. I call out, "Sahaya!" but she doesn't move. She lies facing an old door I found in the rafters of the garage. I attached it to the fence, and called it The Door to Other Worlds. She is cold when I lay my head on her body. She has gone through The Door and left me.

Ruth's husband comes, helps me carry her heavy body into the house, lays her on a soft yellow blanket on my painting table. I'm in a daze. First I clean her carefully. I act without plan or consciousness, find cloth and crow feathers around my studio, make streamers from the cloth. I tie the red cloth strips and black feathers gently on each of her paws, murmuring the little achings of my heart for her to hear. I find a rope of cowry shells, put them around her neck and add a red string of little bells. I want her beautiful when we take her for cremation.

Grief floods everything, and my daughter comes to take care of me. As we come home with the little white box of ashes in my lap, she softly sings a niggun, a wordless, melancholy, sweet tune, in the darkened car. I caress the little white box as though petting a big dog in my lap.

Sahaya lived her name. In Sanskrit her name means beautiful, golden companion. In our time together we radically changed one another. She filled my haven with her articulate silence, yet she was not silent. She spoke to me with sounds, attitude, movement, and intention. She came to understand the languages of my mouth and my energy, and I understood her ways of language. She blossomed into a dog beyond dog. Seeing that, I take courage and think that maybe I can become human beyond human. No words required.

light a candle for Sahaya

she, flying on the night of
balance of light and dark

with red streamers and crow feathers
on her wrists
a braid of cowry shells and bells
round her neck
flying, prancing in her loveliness

they will see her coming.

I can't articulate what it is, but my thinking is still problematic, not just the loss of words. I sit in the cubbyhole office of the neuropsychologist who has been following my progress since the first major problems with my speech here in the West. The desk nearly fills the room. Sitting close, he hands me beautiful little red and white cubes to copy patterns. The task is familiar, but I am straining. He gives me wooden donut shapes to stack in sequences of color and size on little pegs. The time runs out, and I continue on anyway for the solution I know is there. I am oblivious to my scrambling effort. It's only when I get home that I fall apart, can't think, forget that I have a patient waiting for me.

In the third session with the neuropsychologist, I tell him, "I am trying much too hard. After both sessions I've been totally done in! The effort of trying to do well really costs."

"I'm glad you told me this," he says, "I wondered about that; you do put on a really good show of competence. You're trying to mask your difficulties and push on anyway. The testing is showing where your difficulties are."

I am relieved; I want to know the truth; I do want to know the worst.

"It is a little like attention deficit disorder which affects the frontal cortex, distractibility in executive thinking. Only it isn't the same for you." He continues, "Your damage is in the sub-cortex, below the cognitive brain. What you have been experiencing is disorganization at a more basic level than attention deficit disorder. You are having difficulty putting together sensory-body information with perceptual-visual information in your brain. These specific changes are interfering with the organized functioning you want."

I've brooded all these months, the knowing there was something else. What he tells me has the ring of truth. In a practical way I don't get it all, but I see a path forward now.

Taking a walk in the old woods near my house is calming and peaceful. I've come to meditate along the trails, but the green foliage beside me juts out at me in surprise attacks. I can't keep my feet steady. My vision is clear enough, but everything feels blurry. I can't sense the spaces of the dappled woods beyond the path, only the green jumble in my face.

I escape and go to a farmers' market, hoping that talking to a close friend who has a stall there will soothe me. The sunny brightness of the street hammers on my head and the din of happy conversation over flowers and organic peaches cuts into my ears like a buzz saw. Someone jostles me, and I feel barbs all over my body. All I want to do is get out, run away. A trial of medication isn't helping.

On the way to my car, I see Ruth lunching with her husband and his mother at the window table of a Vietnamese restaurant. Impulsively, I go in. I make no small talk to the family, just blurt out to Ruth, "I need a consultation. Could you possibly come by this afternoon?" My voice quavers. Though she is always busy, she says, "Yes, I will come." I know she sees the desperation in my bolt into the restaurant and my agitation. Her husband, and his mother too, see my peculiar behavior. My body relaxes a trifle with the thought she will see me. I pass a vague smile across them all, and rush out. I have to get home to the haven that will enclose this derangement.

When Ruth comes, I've stretched myself on a lawn chaise under the wide canopy of the cherry tree in my backyard in a fitful effort to be comfortable. Just seeing her come through the gate, I am more hopeful, and my body eases.

I hurry to tell her, "I'm very anxious and maybe depressed. I can't sort anything out." She sits down in the white and blue wicker chair near me, leaning close, searches me with her eyes.

"I think you are terribly exhausted," she says. She knows I've been seeing several patients a day, three days a week, spacing them across the day with a day off in between. I thought this strategy would work. "This is too much for you," she says. "Fewer patients, one a day." I'm not happy about this, but I know she is right.

Once again it is brain overload, not anxiety or depression, as I so often think. This is a profound distinction. I have to keep remembering this. I forget so easily. I have been here before, new context, different disability. It was aphasia and loss of words before; now the disability is poor sensory integration and sensory planning. I must pay attention to understanding how these new limitations affect me. Sensory overload is not the same as depression.

In my little garden office, sessions with patients are good; I'm at home in my work. A few weeks later with the new plan, I am not more rested or organized. My life is not easier, and my patients wait weeks between sessions. None of this satisfies me.

I step into my kitchen to clean it up after breakfast. I see dinner dishes piled up for a couple of days. Jars and bags lie around in disarray. Half-sorted mail is all over the table. My body hangs limp on my bones. I'm bleak. I can't see how to straighten up the mess, though I want to.

I am not making art. I walk into my studio and stare at my huge empty painting table. No images ferment in my body now. There is no "Yes!" from core to hands to canvas. Good lord, there is passion everywhere: grief, loss, hope. I feel them all, but the path to act is stunted. I'm mystified. It's like the kitchen; I can't get the wired-in "how-to" to function.

Leigh hears my misery through the phone as we talk one afternoon and says, "Do self-portraits."

"Brilliant idea! So simple!" I reply. It takes me days to manage, because I can't organize myself to get the materials all together easily. Using a mirror to pose myself, I make fast, crude little pencil sketches to get the particular square angle of my jaw, the dark circles around my eyes, and the deep lines around my nose and mouth. Then I make Conté crayon drawings from them, blurred out with water on coarse paper. My mind settles deeply into the coarseness of the texture, the cadged disconnections in my body smooth onto the possibilities of the paper. More drawings and some sketches with paint.

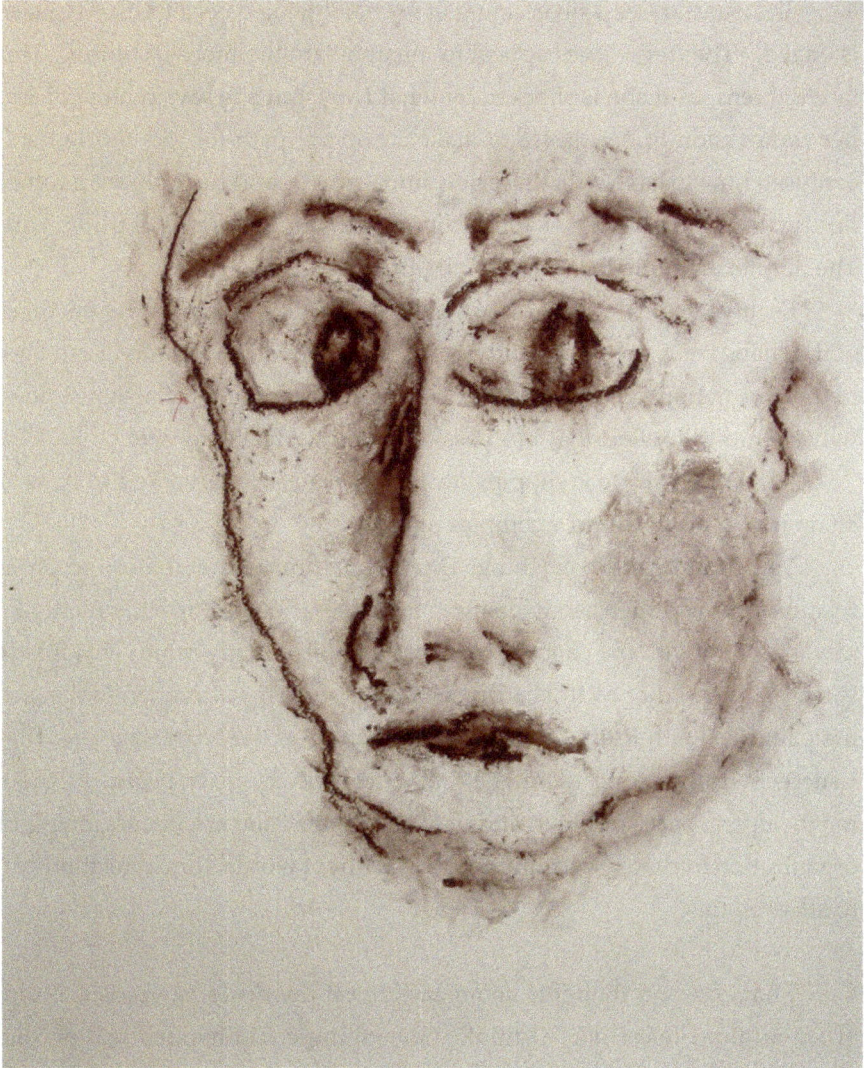

I want the drawings to reveal the ravage I feel. Some feel successful to me; others, shallow. I tack every one of them across the white paneled wall of my studio. I stand and watch them, think about what is true in the whole series as they go up. Ruth looks at them with me and prefers ones that are more idealized and pretty.

"They reflect transformation," she says.

She wants to see a silver lining in my harrowing days, I think. My voice is edged, "The uglier ones appeal to me; they are the more beautiful." Her face tightens, as if she is shocked by what I say, but she says nothing. I feel her compassion in her desire to make a hopeful path for me, but I'm still confused how to cope with these new impairments and can only see another destruction of my life. I look for the hard, dark undercurrents of truth in art. The perplexed numb face I see in my mirror is the art I can do.

Beauty lives in the ugliness of my difficult reality. If I can catch something of the chaos I feel, then I see truth in my condition. That is beauty. I can't get to transformation yet. That isn't the truth now. My living is harsh just now; why shouldn't I reflect that in a passionate way? I feel defensive.

My work, my life is slipping away. The simplicity I worked so hard to attain now feels crushingly complex again.

Yet underneath everything, Oneness supports me, that is, to be in relationship with the vast diversity around me—not a static attainment like nirvana—and with the chaos of creation, now also in my brain. This illness is not an alien-other as it is in dualistic thought. This afternoon looking at the paintings with Ruth, I touch into the depths of the bitter disarray. That I succeeded in making them is a feat, and their diversity begins to show me the open spaces of life in and between them. They are the beginning of organization in chaos, revealing Oneness without words. I am in relationship to all, even this.

I have second thoughts about casting off my doctor's words as I did. "I am afraid. I live alone," I think. "Something could happen and no one would know." I call my daughter and her husband. "If my brains blow up altogether, we do need a plan in place. It is not too soon to think about this. So let's talk."

They agree. "We'll think about it, and get back to you."

I cherish my independence. The quiet of my little carpenter's cottage, the good pleasures of close friends, seeing patients, and my art are the deep comforts in my life. I have the variety, play, and pleasure in the balanced activities that I've carefully constructed for my brain to continue to heal itself. I have the graceful, quiet solitude and luscious, nourishing artwork.

I don't ever want to burden my daughter. My mantra with her has been, "Close but not too close." Enjoy each other, but don't intrude on her life. My mother was cantankerous. After I went to college, we never lived in the same city. Distance was good for me, but not for her. When I visited, she was unhappy, whether I stayed too short or too long. She loved me very much, but her inner irritability walled her tenderness inside it. I don't want any of that with my daughter.

Two days later my daughter calls. "We have independently come to the same conclusion… We would like you to move close to us, sooner rather than later… Before your 'brains blow up,' as you say, we'd like to be able to have some fun time together!"

It is music to my ears. My heart weeps. I'm not my mother. I've feared living out the irascible in my genes. I can have a different way with my daughter, but I can't fully take in the "fun" part.

Not many weeks later I tell them, "It's time. I want to have some of that fun. I'm not having any now. You can start looking for a small house," thinking a year. A scant two weeks later: "We have found a great house for you! Come and take a look."

I'm at the airport with the new downy Satsima, my eight-month-old little service dog, our first flight together. It is pouring rain in a late dark afternoon and we have to trek an unprotected distance across the tarmac. Three planes roar their engines nearby, attacking our ears, and we have to pass them to get to our small commuter plane further out. Satsi, frightened, crouches into the pavement, a sopping golden mop. Though an airline worker carries a big umbrella for us, a high wet wind blows from the side and the thick cloth flaps uselessly in the wet. I lean down to caress the pup, try to soothe him with words to hurry him along. My voice is lost in the noise. I feel as unhinged as the dog.

We are drenched rats stepping into the plane. I think we are boarding first, but I face a cabin full of people already settled. Suddenly I'm hysterical, bitter, and loud. If the plane is not full, there is supposed to be an empty seat next to me, floor space for the service dog. I'm not polite. I'm full of misery. A woman changes her seat for us. The flight attendant tries to soothe me. I don't know how to do this.

The real estate agent is showing me through a '70s ranch-style house. It is all on one level, the way I want. It is plain, efficient, uninteresting. I walk out the back door, and grandeur meets me in the yard. Two grandmother sequoias stand in a magnificent row with a Douglas fir, all towering over me. I am enveloped by their tenderness and grace. I am a stranger here in this yard, and yet my soul rushes to greet their generous spirits. I will buy this house to live beside the roots of these trees.

I put my own sweet little cottage on the market. Family, friends, accountant, financial manager, banker, and real estate agents in both towns all step in to make things happen. They have the how-to I need to get it all done. I sort, give two-thirds of my stuff away to friends, charity, libraries, then box up the rest to move. The effective help of many people makes me feel as though I had a fully functioning brain. Everything flows well, pieces fall into place because of them.

It breaks my heart to close my clinical practice completely. I pictured myself having some amount of professional practice for the rest of my life, like my friend and clinical mentor who was active until two months before she died at ninety. I want that, but my brain tells me it can't do that, no matter what I want. Like other dreams, this one is now gone.

The cottage is empty. I leave a little basket of stones in a corner of the bedroom upstairs. Now I am sweeping down the whole house as my last act of love. As I go from room to room I think of the spirit of the house, how her energy and her calm held and nourished me during these years. Standing now at the front door, I look across the bare living room, through my tearoom and the studio and beyond to a smidge of yard with both sadness and joy. A blessing forms in my mind as a kind of thank-you' I speak aloud to the house as sentient.

Allergic to dust, I sneeze all the way to meet my daughter at the airport near me. She's flown up to drive me, Satsima, my car, houseplants, and last oddments the next distance to my new home.

My one-story house, re-plastered and painted, is sparkly fresh and new for me. I'm starting again, less optimistic, exhausted in my bones. My mind is in rags, over-stretched, full of holes. I pushed my mind beyond itself to scale down, wrap up, and move. Now I sink into a downy cushion of quiet, but so much exhaustion breaks my efforts to put a new face on this future. Despair runs like a hidden stream underneath the losses.

I imagine my daughter and her husband moving into this house to take care of my decline. I think of ways to live in the studio I'm remodeling from the garage—a sleeping cot at the back corner with a paisley throw on it, a tea table in the front window, a couple of wicker chairs for guests, and my painting tables in the center—so I can leave the rest of the house to them. I tell this story to my daughter, and she soothes me off this edge of melancholy.

My life is a shambles … again. I remember I have virtuoso experience. I've lost speech and now other pieces of my mind. I know the elements of rehabilitation: challenge just enough, rest enough, and ensure pleasure in my life. To make new life, I have changed everything before. I can do it … again.

I fill my days working out rehabilitation for this new set of impairments: sensory perceptual planning, strategy, and motor coordination, as the neuropsychologist explained them to me. I set about re-interpreting that information, specifically how the damage affects my life, and then figure out how to challenge different functions of my brain where the damage is—sub-cortical, the cerebellum. I use art and exercise for rehabilitation, as I have done, but now I use them in different ways and to different purposes.

An experienced, supportive yoga teacher helps me to stretch and strengthen my dark body against the fatigue, to begin to revitalize new energy. In Downward Dog posture, I stretch into my arms and then into my legs, asking the muscles to move further, and then rest in Child's Pose for a few moments.

Nia dance exercise classes with my daughter form a major part of my sensory-motor practice. My first class is early morning in her spacious mirrored studio. Satsi lies on his mat near me on a riser, and I stand on the polished dance floor. I'm listening carefully to the music and trying to feel the beat of it in my body at the same time. Even this is hard. The class begins with small stepping movements to the music. I hear the music, feel the beat, make one small movement with my hands; this is the most I can do. I can't do anything more complex than that. I want very much to press beyond my limits into the choreography, step forward and back rapidly, my arms moving up and out, stepping to the side and circling back.

My body weeps that I can't do this and aches remembering how it could be stirred by music, could move lyrically like water to music. To get better I have to stay with the small coordination that I can actually do. I will learn body awareness in motion, blending forms from dance and martial and healing arts. It is a practice based in joy of sensation.

What's in the black box that I imagined at the beginning in the hospital now isn't words or sensory mind, but movement, planning, and sensory coordination. I was an observer in my baby research and in my clinical practice. I use this capacity now. I notice what my failures in daily functioning are and look for activities that will challenge them. Going slowly with the challenges I set for myself is the way to recover. To listen extensively to own my body is new. I start to be aware, in the Nia dancing, of the sensations in the 73 trillion cells, the community, the diversity that makes up my body. I'm a fractal of the larger oneness. I'm in kindergarten again.

The most pleasurable part of my rehabilitation practice is the vision to superimpose my artery images on self-portraits using my new computer and art software. I'm starting new here, too. I first set the computer up on a white Formica table in one of the little bedrooms. In the meantime the building of the studio from the attached garage is progressing. I have a thing for making other uses out of garage space, like my garden office before. When the white-walled studio with high track lighting and two skylights is finished, I move all the art there. The computer and printer go along one wall, my big painting table in the center. There are large windows in the front and side, giving the best light of the whole house.

 I know only the bare basics about computers, and the art software is a mystery to me. Word-to-action sequencing is still difficult, and now I have the additional impairments in sensory planning and work strategies. I can't dream of taking an actual computer class, far too much information to handle. So I find an artist who's willing show me only the one or two steps I want to know. One afternoon I sit with him in his studio and he shows me how to do the five little steps it takes to erase unwanted background from my angiogram x-rays. I ask him to show me again, and yet again. Weeks later I call him to teach me how to resize images.

 I've upped the ante of difficulty considerably to create this artery-portrait. Many times I start over, try again. Like the movement practice, I have to learn one small piece at a time.

 I begin Shotokan Karate for focus, fierceness, and energy awareness, and because the sensei has such a huge, grounded heart, I would follow him anywhere. Karate challenges everything for me. Standing before the dojo, Sensei tells us all, white to black belt, "Presence and intent are essential, not aggression." I stand there in the back row in the middle school gym with the other white belts and wonder at his words. I think that presence and intent are qualities of my mind, but Sensei is saying they are radiant qualities to develop in my body.

 Yoga, Karate, Nia, the computer, and now the addition of games of solitaire are all ruses to urge my brain into flexibility and coordination again. And in their different ways, they give pleasure and variety to my days. Easy speech fluency is gone. I've lost expression again, speak little in groups, even with family around the dinner table. Small chitchat is all I can do. I am invisible again.

 With the stroke, I learned how to balance the damaged verbal left brain with the sensory, creative, expansive right brain. This time, with these different limitations, the route to recovery is listening to the intelligence of my body, the array of sensations that give me information, orientation. Like listening to the landscape of the Pacific Northwest, I learn to listen to the sensory landscape in my body. Pleasure is essential in my healing life again, so that disappointment doesn't follow all the dogged practice. The activities need to be fun to sustain me, to keep me going.

Satsima is fine company and takes care of me in the ways I hoped Sahaya would do, and more. I named him before I met him: Maha Satsima, meaning "a very great good fortune" in Sanskrit. I call him Satsi, but in public he is Handsome Dude. Satsima isn't doggy enough for people to remember.

One night he throws pillows off the couch in the living room, pushing with his head to get my attention because he thinks I'm on the computer too long in the studio. I continue anyway, so he scrapes his front paws on the couch, noisily making a mess of the slipcover. Irritated, I scream at him, but still don't stop. He throws more pillows until, finally, I do stop what I am doing. He is right; I've way overstretched my stamina, as my irritation and screaming show me all too well. Tonight he makes me pay attention to where my limits are.

In a morning Nia class, Satsima is fast asleep on the risers as we are well into the routine. Suddenly he bolts awake, crosses the floor to where I'm dancing, and rubs his head against my leg. He is telling me I should slow down. I see what he has done, and I realize he is right. Another day in a yoga class he lies beside me, he on his mat and I on mine. It is coming to the end of class and I'm thinking of a doing a full bridge. He moves over to my mat and sits on my chest, preventing me from even trying. Acutely sensitive to me, he notices before I do when I overextend my abilities, a great advantage to me in learning how to be more aware moment by moment.

Satsi, beauty on all levels, stands as my front man against my disability and my invisibility. His intelligence is essential to my recovery.

A dream wakes me up suddenly in the middle of the night. In it I am doing a computer search in the university library, and it gives me a title, "Rocks, Fossils, and Flying." Still half-dreaming, I pull the white comforter over my shoulders, dog still lightly snoring at my feet. I muse for a few minutes, intending sleep, but the words nag my consciousness and don't let me. So I get up. Satsima gets up with me and follows me into the studio and lies down on his blue fleece mat beside me. I sit at my computer, thinking and writing.

Rocks and fossils are evidences of a living past. Visions come to me of layers of silt and stone season upon season in ancient streambeds lying far under the surface of today. In my dreamy awake mind I see ancient glaciers scouring the land to bedrock in crushing movements, pushing boulders at their forward edges to distant places. I see the crashing as continental plates collide, their shelves lifting to form mountain chains.

So it is with my life, I think. The scouring of the stroke sheered my edges, polished them brightly, and cleaned out the graveled layers of speech. Sensory materials, their very physicality, form the geologic layering of my life. Layers of my experience are all there under the surface. The geology of me sits here with me this dark morning.

Fossils are like little novellas, telling stories of the immense varieties of plant, animal, and fish that have lived on this planet before this time. There are striking correspondences in body structure and behavior in vastly different species across eons of time. In older human oral cultures, people located themselves deeply in the sensory experience of the intimate relationships of the world around them—trees, mountains, animals, birds, their community.

With the loss of speech, I lost the narrative of verbal planning. Life was much harder in the beginning because the planning, orienting part of language I depended on was a further loss. These two losses eclipsed the primacy of my verbal mind and moved me into a larger narrative. I listen to stories and lives of trees, rocks; I'm in relationship with qualities, spirits, and beings I can't see. These narratives are not verbal, but still they resonate in other parts of my brain as realities.

In archeological time, paradoxically, everything is new and very little is new. Some few basic patterns reconfigure over and over in different life forms across time, creating immense variety. I live at the edge of these ancient processes. I, too, have re-formed and reconstructed. I am comforted by the magnificence of being a part of this vastness, humbled to live as human in the maelstrom of so much diversity.

The coos, jabbers, clucks, knickers, murmurs are among the first oral sensory languages of animals, parents, lovers, and babies, communications full of comfort, vitality, passion, and meaning. The swish of the mountain meadow grasses, the scent of asters and dogwood, each speaks its language.

The trees in my yard murmur and co-breathe with me. They breathe oxygen to me, and I, carbon dioxide to them. It is an intimate and delicate relationship without special agency or thought. The trees talk to one another through roots and pheromones, to the birds that sway in their branches nibbling tiny life in their branch crannies. The luscious scent of my wild roses drags me across my yard.

The din of incessant human words drowns that. The silence I heard after the stroke made hearing these other languages possible. I have been developing a sensory mind all this time. It is wider and deeper than my verbal mind was. Sensory mind belongs to the moment of now and the flow of all the sensory experience of all the others around me and the long eons before my life. The breadth of experience of the trillions of cells in my body sing me alive. Sensations of my family, the soaring trees in my yard, water flying across my sky as white wisps of cloud this morning, the jays and the crows rushing to the feeder next door all are present in my existence this dark morning.

I wonder: What did my body think when my brain no longer processed sensations into emotions? It must have felt loss, and perhaps grief, not in my mind, but in all my sensory tissues. Emotions are not gone; they speak in my body. If I think that everything valuable is in my brain, then my feelings are gone. When I think with my body, the whole sensory array of emotions becomes alive in me. I'm learning to think more with my body, becoming aware of the sensations there that receive the world around me. When I lost speech in the stroke, my body was a barely a partner. With the new basic damage in sensation and perception, I have to understand my body more deeply to recover. My daughter coaches the class in a morning Nia class: "Think of your arms and shoulders as wings and move into free dance." Immediately I feel the muscles in the center of my back and sense that they are large and strong to lift the wings I see in my mind as eagle wings. I perceive directly from my body the sensations of flight as I circle, swoop, and turn. My brain receives the input from my body second.

Feeling the desolation of the young woman muted by stroke and the grief of the older woman losing the clinical practice that was her lifework, I can listen and feel both of them.

To learn the breadth of my non-verbal mind and the depth of what my body can tell me through so much chaos is bittersweet. It's like tasting dark chocolate melting in my mouth.

Deborah Zaslow, storyteller and memoirist, rips each chapter I write to shreds. In her tiny blue handwriting, she creates alternatives around my words. I think about them and write again. The more she rips, the more in love I am.

I've willingly stretched myself out on this rack, yielding to the tearing away of my old language habits. I yearn for renewal. No language is sufficient to tell what it is like inside without words, certainly not the language I knew and lost. I sweat in effort to tauten and compress these vast acres of experience.

For so long I was avid to mediate the loss, so eager to return to some piece of the verbal culture. I ached toward words. I've been torn apart and reconstructed, finding worlds without words, and like a baby, comparing and organizing what is there: perception, sensation. I've come out of the desert again, the black box of words gone. I wonder why I would want to return to the sweltering metropolis of language anyway. I don't want to resume the same somnolent stew, the dispassionate accuracy, the din of barren verbosity.

In the dreamy dark morning I stand at a continental divide, word mind on one side and sensory mind on the other. I think it must be an either/or choice; I haven't lived how to do both at once.

I get back on the rack to stretch and shred my language, to discover a way of expression that I can love. My mind treks in other territories: nerve, fiber, and marrow, searching for the understory of language, voice, song. I wonder how to paint my sensory mind into words so that I can see vividly the inner story I'm trying to tell.

In the original stroke twenty-five years ago, I lost both expressive language and the supporting syntax of daily life activity. The loss of life syntax was language-related: planning, communicating, and executing intent and goals were all affected. In the process, however, I gained art, a mystical mind, and vast non-word relationships in the journey.

In this second event, the damage is to the sub-cortical cerebellum, where some of the most basic integration of sensory-perceptual planning, organization, and implementation of motor activity takes place. From the outside I look reasonably coordinated, but internally I feel off balance and very limited in multitasking across sensory-modalities. And I lost verbal facility again.

I thought that the new damage was not related to the decline of my speech, that my attention went necessarily to the damage of new limitations and only secondarily to my expression. I learn from my neuropsychologist that is only part of the story. The cerebellum is part of the old, primitive brain, the first place where incoming information is organized. As such it provides the most basic direction for both thought and action. So damage in that area of my brain likely limited input into my higher cognitive/verbal brain, accounting for feeling the enormous complexity and the great effort of activities that formerly were simple.

While everything ultimately connects to the brain, my functional disabilities this second time are in my body, motor and somatic, and less in my cognitive mind. The subtle sensorimotor syntax for dancing, for karate, for cleaning my bathroom, and for any other daily life task are now challenges in my body. The sensations of difficulty in sensory-perceptual-motor coordination and syntax in action feel quite different from the consciousness of struggle in cognitive word planning.

The cerebellum, part of the animal mind, provides the basis of sensory thinking. I function best now when I don't think cognitively, when I don't try to figure things out, and allow my body's sensory mind to tell me how to do what I am trying to do. The music of Nia , the rhythm of yoga vinyasas and karate katas all coordinate into body awareness. By paying close attention to the details of movements, I learn how much articulate information my body gives me without words. I'm learning virtually a whole new way of being with my body, gaining awareness of it as a sensing body, being more present to it in the moment.

Over time all my different rehabilitation practices, asking my brain to do this, learn that, the blood vessels, and the communicating nerve fibers together have made a new, larger brain. Challenge and variety create new functional brain. This new brain has altered itself beyond the verbal damage, beyond the sub-cortical damage. I made use of flexibility to change many losses into gains, finding new interests and abilities I hadn't considered before. Once again my life slowly renews from chaos, and as in chaos theory itself, the more complex a system becomes, the more likely a dramatic reorganization will occur.

I restart the clinical practice I thought I would never have again. In this new practice I am pulling together everything I've learned on this harrowing, transforming journey, using the promises of a flexible, plastic brain that can be urged to recover.

Most ordinary people, including professionals, have grown up with the idea that if one has damage to the brain, one is pretty much out of luck, some recovery but not a whole lot. In the 1980s I took for granted that my prospects were limited. I basically paid no conscious attention to that idea, only directly to the limitations in front of me. As it turned out, I saw changes in my expression, easier word finding, better fluency, easier conversation. If I looked back a week, a month, a year, or over many years, I could see progress.

In the meantime there was a major paradigm shift in neurophysiology. While functions in the brain are in fact relatively localized, the brain is understood to be extraordinarily plastic. If there is damage and one tells the brain to function anyway by using therapeutically focused behavior, the brain will use an adjacent area or some other area to do what it is told. That is, the brain can change the real estate. The brain itself is an open, dynamic system, not closed as in the theory of a localized brain.

I didn't know that was happening all these years, but plasticity is precisely what did happen in my brain. I'm a poster woman for neuroplasticity; I'm a 30-year longitudinal observational study, n=1. There is great power in neuroplasticity and considerable hope for change in the neurological status quo.

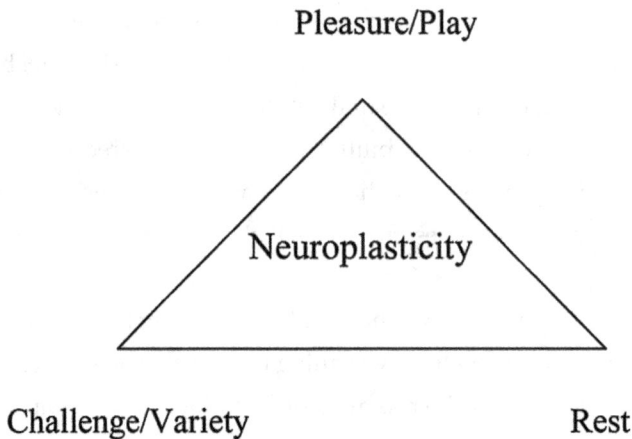

Pleasure/Play

Neuroplasticity

Challenge/Variety   **Rest**

Creating Plasticity, Fig. 1

This is my recovery experience, a model I use in my clinical practice with patients for creating neuroplasticity. It shows how a brain can return to better functioning, how a brain recovers vitality. Fun and varying the input not only make activities therapeutic, they also make rehabilitation more effective in terms of functional gains and speed of recovery.

Stroke and brain traumas create losses in function, in being able to live life well, and add stress and chaos. Rehabilitation strategies are the essential beginning. Art, different kinds of art, dance exercise, karate, computer, solitaire—a motley array—work for my particular condition. I challenge my disabilities one by one, focus activities with practice, practice, practice. I'm certainly desolate at times, but I never give up. I find challenges that feed my soul, give me pleasure and hope in my life.

Far beyond the recovery efforts, I gained treasures in my life that wouldn't have been found but for the loss of speech, powerful ways of expressing and communicating without words.

Personal passions and pleasures are, for me, core conceptions for rehabilitation. Passion gives life personal meaning and, in addition, can be used as incentive and motivation for deepening into successful rehabilitation. My first private practice patient using the model in Figure 1 was a young man with early Parkinson's Disease who had been well maintained on medication for some years. He had given up the two major passions in his life: cross country skiing and piano playing. Explaining the principles of neuroplasticity to him, I urged a return to skiing, starting with retraining his coordination and strength so that he could resume the sport safely. Not only was he a much happier man after a year of training and another year of major cross-country treks, his trunk and head tremors were gone. His hand tremors, being more distal and more difficult to change, nonetheless were significantly reduced after resuming piano practice. He successfully pushed back the progress of the disease and now, in fact, has some personal control over it.

I think often about the question: What happens, in losing speech, to my sense of self? The damaged verbal function affects how ineffective I feel in the world, to be sure. Parallel issues are uncertainty about how much function I can get back and how to construct a life. But most of the time, I see the aphasia and the sensory-perceptual issues as difficulties, just difficulties. For me the presence of significant limitation functions to soften the boundaries of self. I am more permeable to possibility.

I was not in the least talented in art, yet I have become an artist. I was an agnostic and cognitive minded, and I have become a mystic. I have changed the shape of my sense of self. Rather than experiencing the various limitations as alien to self, to be fought against, I see in retrospect that I've used them as stepping stones to reinvent ways to live around and beyond them. My sense of self, rather than collapsing under the weight of catastrophe, which can happen, has become larger and more encompassing, more adventurous, more curious.

From a clinical perspective, I draw a line between my damaged brain and my healthy "regular" brain, knowing that my healthy brain is the residence of my sense of self. I am applying this two-brain idea to how I think about some post-stroke and post-trauma patients that I see in a hospital-based rehabilitation program. Some of these patients believe that the former effective functioning of their brain is gone and therefore think of themselves as different persons. They begin to construct a new sense of self based on the information the damaged brain gives them, begin to act, and think that self-image is true, leaving them with a skewed view of self, world, and future. A middle-aged woman survived a stroke and understood clearly that her brain was impaired. She believed that she had totally lost the brain that she had; then she believed that her husband was having an affair with a former wife and that he would not take care of her after she was discharged. As a clinician, I see the self issue in this patient and others similar to her as a neurological problem and not fundamentally psychiatric. The physically damaged part of this patient's brain was doing the major thinking, giving her garbled information and poor judgment.

I think of this woman as being in a "two-brain" transitional neuro-developmental phase: a damaged brain and a healthy one. In clinical intervention with her I told her she now has two brains and that her old healthy brain was definitely not gone, but that she was listening to the damaged brain far too much and it was giving her wrong information. I asked myself the question: Could I change the balance of her attention from the damaged brain to the healthy one, thus reinstituting the original sense of self? Yes, this patient returned to her original crabby self, but a self with vitality and brass. She began to see and work with the differences between her neurological condition and other issues involved with her discharge plans, and how to think about her future.

In my experience, such patients are relieved, actually, when their sound brain underneath the havoc they are experiencing is affirmed; then they can begin to see the pre-stroke self and hold onto it. Alternatively, another patient who had a cerebellar stroke liked the new, more assertive, aggressive brain and chose to stay with the view of the damaged brain, and began to actualize a changed sense of self.

As a clinician and developmentalist, I see brain recovery processes over time. Patients like me come out of stroke or brain trauma in shock, struggling to sort out what has happened to them, the damages, the limitations. When the dust of shock settles, patients who can begin to work out assessments for themselves. This is a transitional time excellent for informative intervention.

Many of my hospital patients seem almost automatically to opt for the familiar self and work with their limitations as just that, as I managed to do. In the process of this intensive hospital-based rehabilitation, these patients learn the importance of their own activity in their recovery and leave the hospital having learned the basic realities of neuroplasticity. But like the spunky irritable patient described before, many patients struggle with erroneous messages from the damaged parts of their brains. For these patients intervention to assert a shift in attention and awareness from the damaged brain to the familiar can be effective. With that patient I was just as crabby as she while she struggled with me. She knew I had been where she was and therefore trusted my words.

In the time of my stroke and through the following surgery, I was acutely aware of being nearly dead, so close, like a hair's breadth, to being dead, and I survived. To survive such a blow, even with damage and limitation, is an open doorway, a possibility to look at life in a fundamentally different way, to look at purpose and goals anew. Life energy and power reside in that open place. Over time I found totally new perspectives on my life: death became not fearsome but an ally living in my body, paradoxically promoting life, enriching it.

The drawing and painting first were speech therapy, balancing left and right brains, then later the painting became an ecstatic expression of walking a tightrope, balancing life and death in my body. These perspectives are gifts from the fertile space of the stroke experience and disability I wouldn't have otherwise found. My life has richness in it because the stroke and the nearness to death threw me out into different realms of possibility.

As clinician and survivor I often speak to patients about their having survived and its profound meaning for what comes next. A 92-year-old man a few days after a stroke sat up in bed and asked in a fitful voice, "What is the meaning! What is the meaning!"

I replied, "You've survived! You are not dead. That is the meaning. You are alive. This a good thing!" His body relaxed into the bed, and his face became calmer. He had been taciturn all his life, a simple man, a laborer. He becomes talkative after the stroke, speaking magnificently all that he had not said or shared before. His sons and many of his grown great-grandsons were sitting around him there in the hospital room, listening, asking questions. His wife of seventy years was happy with this change, and his great-grandchildren had the pleasures and benefits of hearing his wisdom and his vast experience.

I'm sitting at my computer, pondering these thirty years of personal recovery enduring two different sets of neurological damage. From the larger perspective of my life, I realize I first lost most of my sensory observing mind as a baby in a culture that values words over sensory experience. That is what we do to babies in this culture—help them lose the gift of sensory perception.

Then I lost the verbal mind of the observing psychologist and woman. In that loss I was hectic to find a self I could take out into the world to be seen. And then I lost how to plan, how to move with the music of my body, and how to envision through my body's intelligence. The losses gave me gifts of deeper awareness of myself and of the human condition: the beauty of finding non-verbal languages from loss of language, the perspectives I can articulate from living so long inside loss and disability, the capacity to return to clinical practice once again with those insights and to be of service to patients in a unique way.

As a clinician I am now looking from three perspectives simultaneously: from inside my own experience of stroke; from my long experience as a phenomenological observer, taking theory from what I see; and from the patient's situation, all at the same time. I have become a unique sort of neuro-recovery specialist, a hybrid of phenomenological observation, survivor, clinician, and neuro-developmental educator.

In this long journey I've found a sensory mind and a thinking body. I've not only expanded my brain's functioning, but I've amplified the boundaries of my sense of self. From an abstract mentalist self, I am now a sensate self, a body-experienced self, with a sensory mind.

Today I'm ready to layer the artery images over the self-portraits. I've gotten a new computer and art software to give pleasure, challenge, and immense effort all in one. The crux is play and experiment to create the portrait in my mind's eye. The challenge is to push my lagging capacity to sequence, to coordinate eye and mind, to multitask a complex vision.

I've bought the simplest digital camera to photograph the ugly-beautiful Conté crayon drawings and transfer them to my computer. My new neurologist helps me get my angiogram x-rays onto CD, but once in the computer they lose the transparency of film. I struggle bit by bit to learn exactly, and no more, the pieces of program I need to make this complex layered image I see in my mind.

I'm irritable, push my limits, seek patience, hope for beginnings of skill. The vision I hold of the portrait and the process of getting to it, they are my pleasures—and my defeats.

I sit in my new studio with skylights casting soft light into the room. I'm keyed up, tense. I start in one place, fumble through a nightmare maze of unfamiliar program variables, fall into black holes, and wind up in another place.

It's a mess ... I take a mental step back and ... look again ...

It is stunning, this portrait. The artery moves over the face like a river running tributaries. The face has no mouth; one eye penetrates the viewer and the other gazes ....

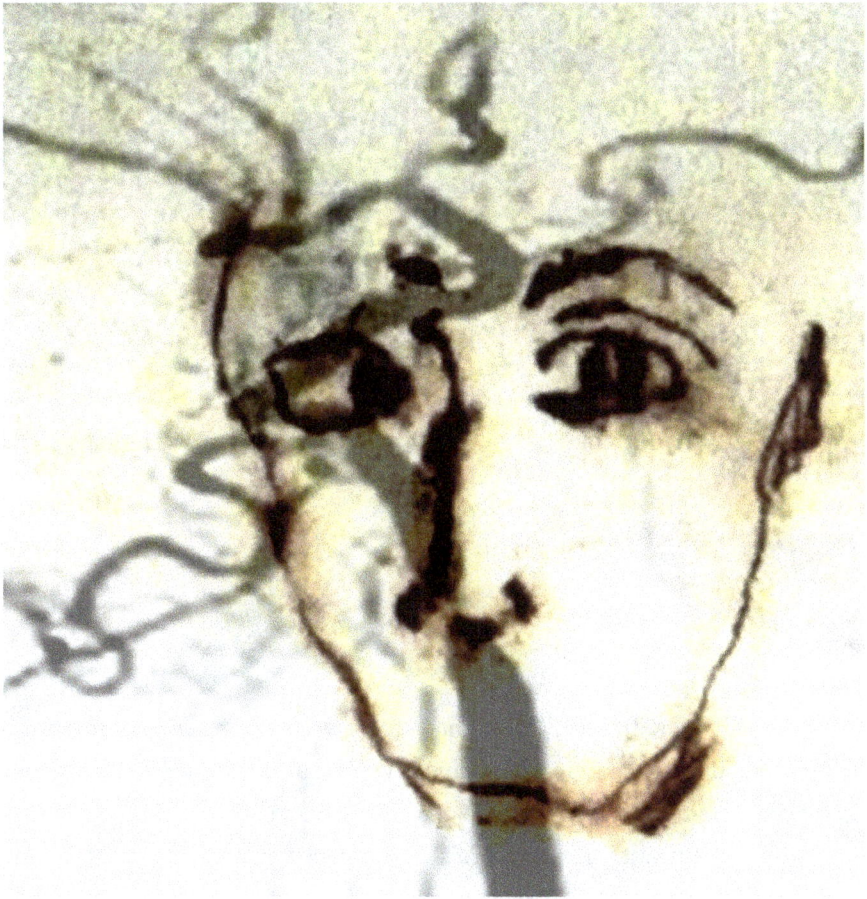

.... into another world. It isn't the image I had in mind; it's scope is far larger. The portrait affirms magnificence.

Now, now I can see transformation.

My life too is messy, surprising, and … stunning.

I make more portraits, counting on mess and happenstance. I like what I see. They are awesome in their strangled, painful beauty. I make abstractions from the patterns my vessels make, playful, alive.

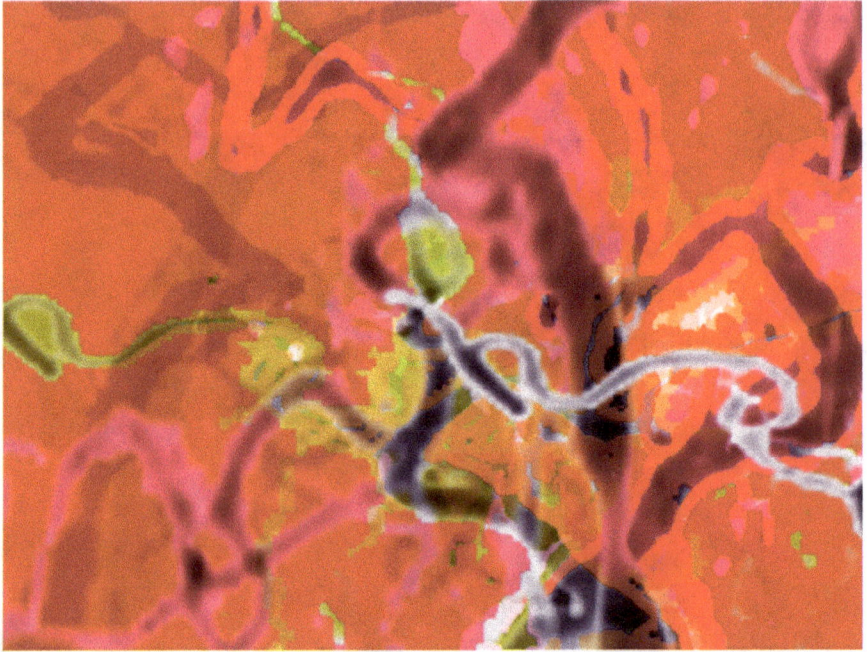

Art is like meditation. I don't have to be talented or strive for nirvana. I simply practice and practice what gives me pleasure, anything that will hone in on challenging my hurt brain.

I feel the beauty of the vessels in the portraits crossing my face and inside my head know their awesome flexibility in my life. They have moved through the tissues in my brain, reshaped their space, and gone where there was need. The vessels nourished the damaged tissues of my brain to make new brain.

I was alone when I was without words, and then I was blown through a doorway by my heart with love for my daughter. In the company of so many others, material and non-material, I have moved in non-word places. Without the landscape of utterance, I've unearthed treasures, wreathed and adorned myself with an extravagance of sensory languages. Dressed in them, I've gone to the heart of what is … and pressed toward the edges of what can be. I've moved in spaces where mystery collides with mind and melts into vision.

Beginner's mind is here now. Sensory experience is now. Perception is now.

No words required.

Appreciation

Many path makers gave me road signs on the way out from the stroke. The ones named: Jake Yake, Dr. Martha Sarno, Dr. Katherine Smith z'il, Dr James Correll z'il, Dr. Yehuda Nir, Robert Bly, Henry Pearson z'il, Leigh Kimball, Dr. Ruth Chaffee, Deborah Zazlow.

Many many unnamed are as blessed for me in the journey as the named. Those who could see me when I was invisible and could hear me when I could say so little.

My first flower drawing teacher is nameless because the stroke wrecked remembering proper names. She was the pointer to my seeing the unique in how I see and to sending me to Henry Pearson and thus to my becoming a painter.

To unpack what happened in the Lakota ceremony, I studied with David Spangler, modern mystic, for decades, learning and practicing subtle activism in the Lorian community. Rabbi Aryeh Hirschfield, z'il, practiced the mystical publicly. He talked to the Mystery; I could see and feel it around me. He showed me not only a mystical Judaism but also a Judaism that reaches outward and embraces all belief, could embrace the Christian Jewish agnostic me. It was Rabbi Marc Sirinsky who brought all of that into the bare bones of my life shattering the walls of isolation, love and creativity

Vision makers: Aaron Ortega, Shotokan Sensei . . . . Stephen Victor, Fields of Grace, constellation work…..also adepts in their paths and deep lovers of life. Paul Richards' energy work after the chaos of brain trauma., reorganized everything and perhaps extended my life.

Dr. Oliver Sacks' work was the profound inspiration for my doing this story as an inner narrative, and maybe for doing it at all.

Rachael Resch and Richard Seidman's part in this story is dim compared to the brilliance they are in my life. Rachael is center in the whole of my life story: her wisdom, her beauty, her creativity with her life, her own prodigious capacity for endurance. Richard loves my daughter, and what mother doesn't love a man for that. He quietly tends the world we live in, profoundly touches lives around him in deep and important ways, including this memoir. Both of them shared their wisdom and time far beyond generosity for me and this book.

The subtext of resilience in the story had a mentor before the narrative. Dr. Cecilia Karol was my psychoanalyst. From the dark mine of my unconscious and the wishes of my life, she sturdied me so that I could deliver on my dreams through the chaos that came after.

Editors and writing teachers: Deborah Zazlow first, then Marc Sirinsky, Jay Shroeder, Richard Seidman, Austin Rachlis, Fayegail Bisaccia, and David Zazlow. Robert Jaffee photographed some of my early art work and is the stellar printer for my limited edition giclee prints. PJ Florin did diligence over and over proofing the details of my written language.

And last and first my dedicated and devoted publisher, Jeremy Berg.

It takes a village to blossom a writer . . . thank you!

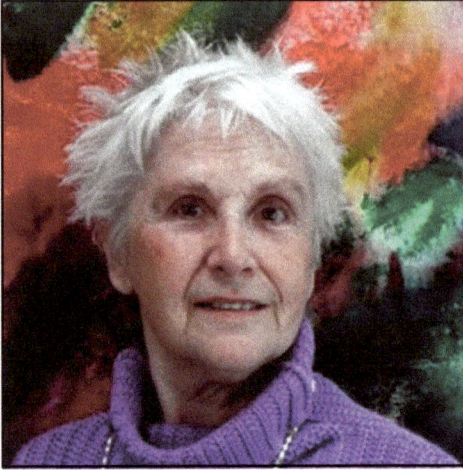

Ruth Resch is a clinical psychologist, gifted by random chaos to become an artist, writer, and poet. She lives in the Pacific Northwest with Handsome Dude, her Service Dog, who keeps her in line.

Photo by Marc Sirinsky

Contact Information:

www.withoututterance.com
www.ruthresch.com
withoututterance@jeffnet.org

Media Kits
may be downloaded at www.withoututterance.com or by inquiry at withoututterance@jeffnet.org.

Information and Inquiries for Talks and Professional Consultations through the websites or email.

Orders and Wholesale Orders
lorianpress@msn.com

www.ingramcontent.com/pod-product-compliance
Lightning Source LLC
Chambersburg PA
CBHW072250270326
41930CB00010B/2339